Applied Occlusion

Quintessentials of Dental Practice – 29
Prosthodontics – 5

Applied Occlusion

By

**Robert Wassell, Amar Naru,
Jimmy Steele, Francis Nohl**

Editor-in-Chief: Nairn H F Wilson
Editor Prosthodontics: P Finbarr Allen

Quintessence Publishing Co. Ltd.
London, Berlin, Chicago, Paris, Milan, Barcelona, Istanbul,
São Paulo, Tokyo, New Delhi, Moscow, Prague, Warsaw

British Library Cataloguing in Publication Data

Applied occlusion. – (Quintessentials of dental practice; v. 29)
1. Occlusion (Dentistry)
I. Wassell, Robert II. Wilson, Nairn H. F.
617.6'43

ISBN-13: 9781850970989

ISBN-13: 978-1-85097-098-9

Foreword

Just when you thought that the *Quintessentials of Dental Practice* series had little more to offer, this latest, somewhat larger than normal, volume breaks new ground. The innovation is the inclusion of a fantastic DVD, which brings occlusal concepts and techniques to life, animating and otherwise complementing the excellent text. As a consequence, what other authors have taken many tens of thousands of words to convey, the authors of this book have successfully presented in the succinct format characteristic of the *Quintessentials* series.

Numerous high-quality illustrations, many of which link text and DVD, highlight the immediate practical relevance of the refreshingly pragmatic but robust approach the authors adopt in the management of occlusion in clinical practice.

Knowledge and understanding of occlusion underpins good clinical practice. Without such knowledge and understanding, procedures that change the way teeth function and relate are fraught with risks of iatrogenic damage, let alone being inconsistent with good patient care. If your knowledge and understanding of modern approaches to occlusion are in any way suspect, then this book and accompanying DVD will address this problem, offering superb value for money.

In common with all the other books in the now extensive – more than 40 volumes – *Quintessentials* series, this text is intended to have wide appeal, spanning the broad spectrum of undergraduate student through to experienced practitioner. I can, therefore, encourage clinicians at all levels to add this book to their library, both for detailed study and to be kept to hand for ready reference. An added attraction is that elements of the accompanying DVD may find application in educating patients as to the nature and possible solutions of occlusal problems.

The authors of this volume are to be congratulated on reaching new heights in the literature pertaining to occlusion. In unreservedly recommending this book, together with its accompanying DVD, I am confident that everyone who reads and views the material, so carefully crafted by the authors, will undoubtedly learn and be able to put into practice good occlusal assessment and management.

Another outstanding addition to the highly acclaimed *Quintessentials* series.

Nairn Wilson
Editor-in-Chief

Introduction

This book acknowledges the importance of adopting a clinical approach to understanding occlusion, which can be a difficult subject to understand. We all know it is there and important, but, as it is difficult to visualise, it can sometimes be hard to appreciate this importance. Dentists, whatever their background, will have different perspectives as to how occlusion affects their clinical practice. The authors, a general practitioner (AN), a restorative consultant (FSN) and two senior academics (JGS and RWW), have integrated their knowledge and experience to emphasise the common ground. To keep the book a manageable size we have restricted its scope to teeth, implants and fixed restorations.

Rather than start with some dry definitions, we have considered a number of situations in which the occlusion causes damage to teeth or restorations: damage that is invariably caused by occlusal instability or parafunction, or both. For all of the theoretical occlusal concepts that have been written about over the years, damage from occlusion is what actually matters. In many cases this is iatrogenic. A good dentist needs to know how to detect, treat and avoid such problems.

To describe how the occlusion is associated with day-to-day problems, we have explained and illustrated the possible underlying mechanisms, gradually introducing the reader to important occlusal concepts and definitions. Dr Naru's three-dimensional computer animations together with the narrated clinical movie sequences bring these to life.

We often think of occlusal damage affecting restorations, teeth, supporting tissues and the masticatory system, but, as described in Chapter 1, occlusion can also be damaging for a practice. Think of the situation, which happens all too commonly, when a crown takes hours, or what seems like hours, to fit. Attention to detail with impressions, jaw records, articulation and provisional restorations is needed to prevent such frustration. The development of good practice in all of these areas will benefit any dentist wanting to expand their clinical knowledge and expertise in occlusion.

Chapters 2 and 3 focus on the effects of function and parafunction, respectively. Normal function can damage vulnerable restorations, but poorly contoured restorations can interfere with function, which further increases the risk of damage. Parafunction involves large forces that can wreak havoc, both on teeth and on restorations. Chapter 4 gives advice on conforming with or reorganising an occlusion.

Chapters 5, 6 and 7 explore special considerations of occlusion relating to the periodontium, the provision of implant restorations and temporomandibular disorders (TMDs). It is widely recognised that the majority of TMDs do not have an occlusal aetiology. Nevertheless, there are times when occlusal factors are very relevant, and dentists need to know how to identify and manage them.

The final chapter, Chapter 8 (in 12 sections), is the longest in the book. It contains details of various occlusal techniques, including occlusal examination, recording jaw relationships, articulator choice, diagnostic waxing, copying anterior guidance, occlusal splints and occlusal adjustment.

About the DVD

How many occlusion students have been baffled by two-dimensional diagrams of mandibular positions and movements? With software used to create blockbusting films, Dr Naru has skilfully provided an animated three-dimensional perspective. In conjunction with Chapter 2, he illustrates the importance of anterior guidance, both in terms of normal movement and what can happen when restorations interfere with guidance. With Chapter 3, he demonstrates the problems associated with deflective contacts and interferences.

We have also filmed a number of clinical sequences, beginning at Chapter 7, where we show a structured examination for diagnosing TMDs. In Chapter 8 we use a clinical case of occlusal derangement to illustrate all the clinical and laboratory stages involved in occlusal analysis and occlusal adjustment. This section includes details of how to carry out an occlusal examination and tips on recording accurate impressions, centric jaw and facebow registrations. After considering semi-adjustable and average-value articulators, we move on to mounting casts, trial adjustment and clinical occlusal adjustment. Many of these procedures are common to the management of patients needing extensive restorations or suffering from occlusally related problems.

The clinical case of occlusal derangement shown in the DVD is somewhat unusual in its aetiology, apparently resulting from tooth movements during pregnancy. It is also relatively challenging. Nevertheless, it usefully illustrates the sequence of events common to the management of many occlusal problems.

How to Use the Book and DVD

To guide the reader, Chapters 1 to 7 concentrate on providing an understanding of occlusion, while Chapter 8 concentrates on occlusal techniques. Some may wish to read the book conventionally, starting at the beginning and working through sequentially to the end. Others, confronted by a clinical problem, may wish to read the relevant background from Chapters 1 to 7 and then cross-refer to Chapter 8 for relevant techniques.

The parts of the book complemented by the DVD have headings marked with the DVD logo. In Chapters 1, 2 and 3, many of the figures comprise key frames from the DVD animations. We have marked these with a coded DVD logo, enabling the reader to focus on the animation relevant to that part of the text. Of course, readers may want to get an overview of all the animations as a continuous sequence before reading the book, returning to focus on those areas that need to be reviewed. This is probably the most efficient way to get an understanding of jaw movement and occlusal theory. Therefore, the DVD animations menu has a "play all" button.

There is a separate DVD menu for the clinical videos associated with Chapter 7 and sections of Chapter 8. Again, you can play all the videos as a continuous sequence, but they run for longer than the animations, at just under an hour. Therefore, depending on how you prefer to study, you may wish to view the relevant video either before or after reading these chapters.

Disclaimer

Whilst many occlusal procedures are quick and easy to do, provided the dentist has the required knowledge and skill, some can be relatively difficult and time consuming. Using a bicycle analogy, you may straighten a buckled wheel simply by adjusting one or two spokes. However, all of the spokes may need adjustment or the wheel may have to be rebuilt, demanding considerably more proficiency. We encourage clinicians to develop their expertise, but urge caution when extending outwith their comfort zone; when in doubt, seek advice, or refer appropriately rather than risk irreversible damage and the possibility of patient complaints.

The techniques and principles described in the book are to the best of our knowledge examples of good practice; however, the authors and publishers disclaim responsibility for their application or misapplication.

Acknowledgements

We are extremely grateful to Prestige Dental UK and Waterpik Inc for sponsoring the production of the DVD, and for the support of Newcastle Dental Hospital and School in providing the facilities. Thanks also for the enthusiasm and expertise of all those involved in making it happen: Steve Thorpe for his excellent camera work; Steve Hogg for the many hours spent producing, directing and editing; Lois Lane for the animation voice-over; Kevin Dick and Roger Pusey for the sound recording; dental nurses Liz Smith and Claire Anthony-Mote for their help and patience with the project; Alyson Cooper for deftly accomplishing the technical work; and Mark Siddoway from Newcastle University's Knowledge House for skilfully organising the contractual arrangements. The project would not have been possible without the cooperation and involvement of our patients, to whom we are especially thankful. We also gratefully acknowledge our individual mentors (they know who they are!), who provided the foundations on which we have built our concepts of applied occlusion.

We gratefully acknowledge figures from other publications:
Figs 8-17 and 8-50 to 8-54 reproduced from *Dental Update* (ISSN 0305-5000), by permission of George Warman Publications (UK) Ltd.

Fig 8-60 reproduced from the *British Dental Journal* by permission of the Editor, Stephen Hancocks.

Contents

Contents of the DVD

Understanding Jaw Movement Animations
A. Intercuspal Position (ICP)
B. Lateral Excursion into ICP Showing Disclusion
C. Canine Guidance and Group Function
D. Tracks of Posterior Movement
E. Crowning and Anterior Guidance
F. Protrusive Interference on Crown
G. Retruded Contact Position and ICP
H. Last Tooth in the Arch Syndrome
I. Cross Arch Pivot

Clinical and Laboratory Sequences
J. TMD Examination
K. Occlusal Examination
L. Accurate Alginate Impressions
M. Centric Relation Registration
N. Facebow Record
O. Semi-adjustable and Average Value Articulator
P. Mounting Casts
Q. Occlusal Analysis
R. Trial Occlusal Adjustment
S. Clinical Occlusal Adjustment and Follow-up

The DVD is produced in 4:3 format.

Chapter 1
The Intercuspal Position and Dentistry

Aim

The aim of this chapter is to define intercuspal position (ICP) and its importance to both patients and dentists.

Outcomes

By the end of this chapter, the clinician should:
- appreciate relevant aspects of the physiology and development of ICP
- realise how ICP can be compromised, and the consequences of this
- understand the dental and financial consequences of fitting a restoration that does not conform to ICP, and understand how to avoid this scenario.

Introduction

For all of the complexity of the masticatory system, the most basic occlusal concept is very simple indeed: the top and bottom teeth need to meet together in a way that will allow food to be chewed and swallowed. ICP is the term we will use to describe the position in which the teeth are maximally meshed together. When a restoration is carved or shaped it is usually to conform to ICP. ICP is also the position on which orthodontic classifications are based. Clench your own back teeth together now and you have it (Fig 1-1). You can see how the teeth move into ICP on DVD animation A.

Some dentists call this position "centric occlusion", but we prefer to avoid this term as it means different things to different people. It can also cause confusion with the term "centric relation", which is an important but very different concept (described in Chapter 3). Centric relation is determined by the temporomandibular joints (TMJs) but ICP is determined by the positions of the teeth, and because the two do not usually coincide the difference is important.

In this and the following chapters we will consider occlusally related damage. Damage from problems with ICP is often iatrogenic, the most familiar example being the damaging consequences of providing a high restoration.

1

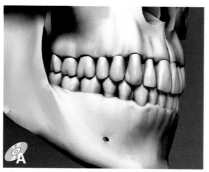

Fig 1-1 Teeth maximally meshed together in ICP.

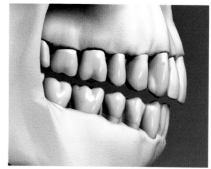

Fig 1-2 Most of the time the mandible is in the rest position with the teeth separated by 2–4 mm, termed "freeway space".

Before looking at clinical problems and ICP, we will provide relevant background regarding its physiology and development. If you are interested in learning more, then the Further Reading section at the end of the chapter suggests appropriate material.

Physiology of ICP

Physiologically, ICP is the relationship of the mandible to the maxilla when the teeth reach the end of the chewing cycle. It is here, at the most closed position of the mandible, that the teeth apply maximum force. It is here that the teeth have closed through the food bolus to break up the food into smaller pieces, and it is also here that the mandible is stabilised, allowing swallowing to take place.

The bony architecture of the skull directs masticatory forces down the long axes of the teeth and into the robust base of the skull. This is a biomechanical triumph with various buttresses and arches transmitting crushing stresses without structural damage. Consider the forces involved in crunching through a nut kernel or breaking up tough fibres of meat – forces endured (incidentally) not only by the teeth, periodontium and bones, but also by restorations. Unlike in a simple nutcracker, however, there is a sensitive feedback system to regulate the amount of force applied to the teeth by the jaw muscles. Typically, forces will:

- vary between 350 and 700 N (10 N approximates to 1 kg) for the maximum biting force

- be about one-third of this during chewing
- be several times higher in the molar than incisor regions.

The neuromuscular system which regulates these forces and jaw movements relies on proprioceptive input from the periodontal ligaments, the tooth pulps, the TMJs, muscles, tendons and ligaments. The periodontal ligament in particular is exquisitely sensitive, able to detect materials between the teeth down to 20 μm – half the thickness of a human hair – a fact worth remembering when placing and adjusting restorations. Also of direct clinical relevance is the potential for feedback from the pulp, predisposing root-treated teeth to higher forces as there is clearly no such feedback. This may partly explain the increased vulnerability of root-treated teeth to fracture.

Not only does the neuromuscular system regulate occlusal forces, it also programmes the muscular activity required to direct the teeth precisely into ICP without conscious effort. The frequent activity of swallowing constantly updates the neuromuscular system so that the muscles can position the mandibular teeth straight to ICP. This programming is impressive, but can make it difficult for the clinician to find and record other relationships of the mandible, such as centric relation. The muscles may need to be "deprogrammed", as described in Section 8-4.

Although ICP is a fundamental concept in occlusion, paradoxically it is not a position held by the teeth for much of the time. Assuming we are in a reasonably relaxed state of mind, classical estimates are that the teeth only come together in ICP for 17.5 minutes a day, comprising approximately 1800 chewing strokes and 500 swallowing contacts. At other times the mandible is at rest, leaving a gap of a few millimetres between top and bottom teeth (Fig 1-2). It is perhaps not surprising then that the prolonged heavy contacts of parafunctional grinding and clenching are potentially damaging.

Development of ICP

During occlusal development in childhood and adolescence, the moulding action of the tongue, cheeks and lips guides the erupting upper and lower teeth into position. In ICP, there appears to be a balance between the eruptive force of the teeth and the day-to-day masticatory forces. If a tooth erupts into a premature contact, it is subject to greater occlusal forces than the adjacent teeth, resulting in its orthodontic realignment. When a tooth is extracted, the balance is lost, accounting for the overeruption, tilting or rotational movements of adjacent and opposing teeth.

Another mechanism which may compensate for uneven occlusal contact is for the mandible to find a new ICP, such that occlusal loads are more comfortably spread. The neuromuscular system will then programme the mandible to find and consolidate this new ICP. This process is probably very gradual and likely to be the reason for the usual discrepancy between centric relation and ICP, although the evidence for this is empirical. Despite these adaptive processes, an even ICP is not guaranteed and some people have anterior (Fig 1-3) or posterior open bites.

Even in adulthood, ICP is not stable over the long term. As teeth wear (Fig 1-4), are restored or lost, the relationships of the upper and lower teeth inevitably change, albeit very slowly and in a way that maintains stability and health. For example, there is slow but continued alveolar growth through life, which is thought to compensate for occlusal wear. Occasionally though, the ICP can "collapse" more rapidly, with loss of vertical dimension and drifting of teeth (Fig 1-5). This is only likely to happen when occlusal support is severely compromised by a lack of supporting teeth, loss of periodontal

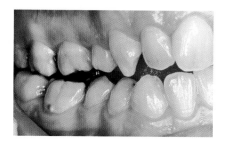

Fig 1-3 Patients often adapt to open bites, but sometimes they cause discomfort and functional problems when they arise later in life.

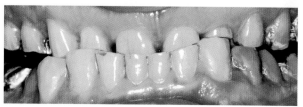

Fig 1-4 Tooth wear is a natural process to which patients normally adapt. However, this patient had excessive wear of his anterior teeth caused by a tooth grinding habit. He had adopted a protrusive posture as his posterior teeth no longer provided stable occlusal contacts.

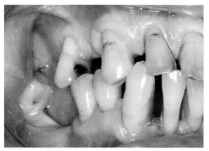
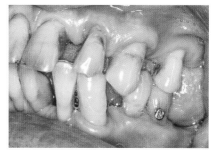

Fig 1-5 Occlusal collapse in a patient with periodontal disease and multiple missing posterior teeth. Notice the splaying of the upper incisors.

attachment or spacing. It tends to occur when these conditions are combined with a significant skeletal discrepancy between the mandible and maxilla (severe Class II or III). Look at Figs 5-5 and 5-7 in Chapter 5 for examples of periodontally related problems.

Finally, a relatively unusual cause of occlusal instability in the natural dentition is the "scissor bite", where the upper posterior teeth lie buccal to the lower. The lack of firm occlusal stop results in continued eruption and often occlusal problems (see Fig 1-6).

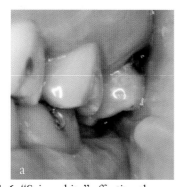
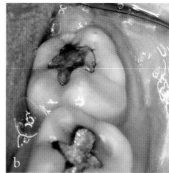

Fig 1-6 "Scissor bite" affecting the upper third molar.
(a) Buccal view and (b) occlusal view of lower molar showing marked wear caused by the palatal cusp of the upper molar overerupting and interfering with jaw movement due to a lack of a firm occlusal stop.

Is There an Ideal Occlusion?

While textbooks have promulgated the concept of "ideal" or so-called "normal" occlusion, it is worth bearing in mind that there is no such thing as a morphologically correct or incorrect ICP. All of the orthodontic "classes" are relatively common, and even Class I relationships are rarely perfect. There are so many normal variations that are completely consistent with adequate function and health that the concept of "correctness" is probably not very helpful. It is normal to be imperfect. Nevertheless, given the pattern of contacts seen in an "ideal" (Class I) occlusion, such that cusps in one arch fit into fossae or onto marginal ridges in the other, it is helpful to define what we try to achieve when providing restorations.

Providing Dental Treatment and ICP

The positions and shapes of the teeth define ICP. In most people, the cusps of posterior teeth in one arch fit into fossae and onto marginal ridges on the opposing arch in a unique way, just as a key fits a lock, providing an ICP that is highly reproducible and stable. Often there will be some, albeit limited, freedom for the mandible to move a little and still maintain contact around the arch. A few people cannot find a single stable position, because of the way their teeth are arranged. This can be uncomfortable and can make dentistry difficult, but is also quite unusual. For most of us, if we close our teeth together we always end up in ICP, smoothly, time and again.

The fundamentally important point about ICP is that, because it is tooth determined, it is only a consistent and stable position if there are enough teeth to define it. If there are no teeth, or if most of the tooth surfaces are removed, for example by preparing them for extensive restorations, ICP will be lost. When making complete dentures, this is what confronts the dentist on every occasion.

On rare occasions when the occlusion needs to be reorganised, for example if the vertical dimension is to be increased, we have to provide a new stable ICP using the teeth that are there, using a range of clues to guide us. In the dentate, this approach is important, technically demanding, but used sparingly (see Chapter 4).

Usually, though, life is simpler; only a few teeth need to be restored at any one time, and so when treatment is provided (e.g. a filling, crown, bridge or partial denture) we can conform to the existing ICP. Conforming is not difficult, but the consequences of getting it wrong are significant and familiar to every dentist (and to many patients). These consequences are best captured by the concept of the "high" restoration.

The High Restoration

Restorations that are left high tend to cause considerable problems to dentists and patients. Of the countless restorations placed every day, it is unlikely that all will be contoured to hair's-breadth accuracy. Clearly, some will be left high. While some patients will ignore a high restoration and may eventually adapt to it or wear it down, others will not.

For patients, a high restoration is a matter of discomfort or inconvenience. To the dentist, it is a matter of professional pride, and money. Few dentists will knowingly allow a patient to leave the surgery with a restoration that is high in ICP because they know that in all probability it will subsequently cost them time and, as a consequence, money. The patient may well return complaining of pain (usually as tenderness to percussion, but sometimes headaches, muscle soreness or TMJ pain) or the restoration will break, a cusp will fracture, or there may be tooth mobility and drifting. None of these consequences are good for building up a practice.

Carving or shaping a plastic filling before it is set is relatively straightforward. By contrast, the time spent repeatedly marking, removing, adjusting and replacing a crown, bridge or onlay can be maddening as the profitability of the exercise evaporates with every turn of the bur. Given that accurate materials are being used by skilled dentists and technicians, the restorations coming back from the laboratory should only ever need the minimum of adjustment, but this is not necessarily the case.

The key to avoiding a laboratory-made restoration being high is to understand why it happens in the first place. It is invariably human error at one or more of the following stages:

- **The working impression:** This is not a likely source of occlusal error. Accurate materials and strong adhesives are available which do not normally allow the impression to pull away from the tray. Flexibility of the tray can occur with very viscous materials such as a putty, but, although this affects the die, the effect on occlusal accuracy is likely to be small.
- **The opposing impression:** Often something of an afterthought, the opposing impression has the potential to be the source of considerable

occlusal error. Gross distortions of the impression where it pulls away from the tray are common. They result in casts that look fine, but which simply do not articulate properly. Section 8-2 has a detailed description of the simple steps to be taken to avoid this and other errors in alginate impressions.

- **The occlusal record:** Although a wax or silicone record may make the dentist feel secure, there is a significant risk that a wax or silicone record may stop the casts from coming into full contact in ICP. Often it is best not to use an occlusal record at all, or to use one that is trimmed and limited only to the preparations, if the ICP is not particularly stable. Section 8-3 describes the technicalities of making the record in more detail.
- **The laboratory handling of casts:** Following removal of the impression, dental casts often have little "blebs" of stone on the occlusal surfaces. These are the result of small air bubbles or voids in the impression. Good impression technique will minimise but not eliminate these. A bleb 1 mm high on an occlusal surface can create a similar space between mounted casts, and 1 mm of excessive occlusal gold takes a lot of grinding. The responsibility for "flicking" off such blebs lies with the laboratory, but it is worth the dentist checking the casts when they have come back to the surgery and giving feedback, as appropriate, to the laboratory.
- **The mounting of the casts:** This has to be done with great care. It is not uncommon for casts to move slightly during mounting. The use of plasterless articulators is fairly common, as they are quick and convenient, but the risk of inaccurate mounting is quite high as the casts often move as the articulator is tightened. This stage is mostly about care and attention to detail. Provided the casts are properly mounted, there should not be a problem in constructing the restoration to fit precisely in ICP.
- **The provisional crown:** If the provisional restoration is poorly formed or lost, overeruption and drifting will result. This will cause not only a high crown, but also an ill-fitting one with tight proximal contact(s).

None of the steps to avoid these problems is time consuming or difficult, but attention to important detail can make a fundamental difference.

Occlusal Stability in Restorations

New contacts are likely to be most stable where a cusp fits into a fossa or where it meets a marginal ridge. In contrast, new contacts are unstable if placed precariously on a cusp slope (Fig 1-7). This may not always be important, but it can have real consequences in the long term because, without stable contacts to hold their positions, teeth can tilt, rotate or overerupt over time. This is a particular problem where there are only a few opposing teeth in the first place.

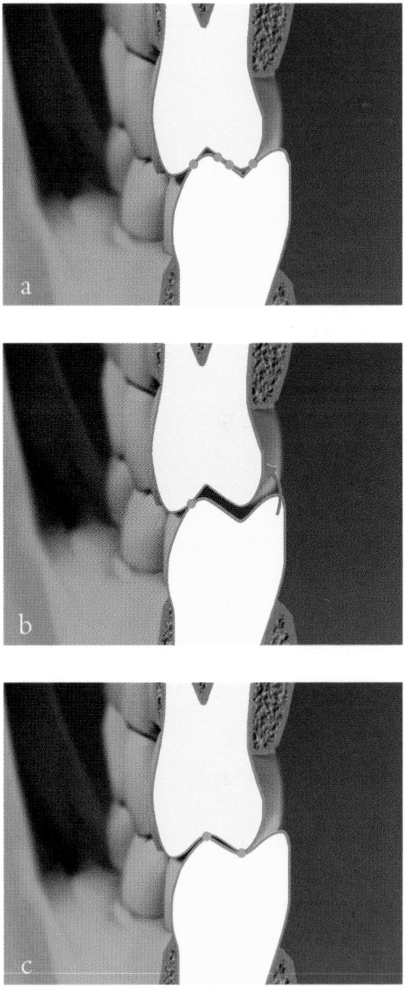

Fig 1-7 Establishing stable ICP contacts in restorations.

Fig 1-7a Stable contacts formed against opposing cusp slopes – a pattern often seen in the natural dentition.

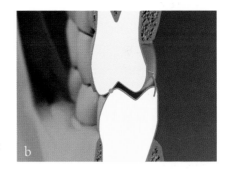

Fig 1-7b Contact formed against a single cusp slope, potentially allowing unwanted tilting and overeruption.

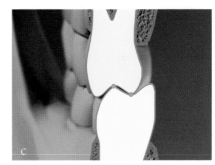

Fig 1-7c Stability may be obtained simply by cusp to fossa contacts.

Why Not Leave Restorations out of Contact?

It is, of course, possible to leave a restoration "low"; in other words, out of contact. This certainly guarantees against some of the short-term consequences of a high restoration. Some dental laboratories may even use a spacer when constructing crowns to ensure that the prosthesis remains out of contact, thus saving the time and expense of adjustment – "carve them low, let them grow".

The use of strategies which deliberately leave restorations out of contact are not sensible. The restored tooth and the opposing teeth are subject to overeruption and drifting. Minor overeruption, rotation or tilting may not be very important in the general scheme of things, but this is unpredictable and unnecessary and can lead to the disruption of excursive tooth contacts or the introduction of premature contacts, risking other problems at a later stage. If this practice is used for multiple crowns, it may severely destabilise the occlusion. Given that, with a little care and attention, it is possible to construct restorations which fit precisely to ICP, the use of strategies to leave restorations out of contact should be redundant.

Conclusion

An understanding of ICP is fundamental to successful restorative practice and to understanding all of the more complex aspects of dynamic occlusion.

Further Reading

Ash MM, Nelson SJ. Wheeler's Dental Anatomy, Physiology, and Occlusion. St Louis: Saunders, 2003:437–489.

Fennis WM, Kuijs RH, Kreulen CM, Roeters FJ, Creugers NH, Burgersdijk RC. A survey of cusp fractures in a population of general dental practices. Int J Prosthodont 2002;15:559–563.

Gragg KL, Shugars DA, Bader JD, Elter JR, White BA. Movement of teeth adjacent to posterior bounded edentulous spaces. J Dent Res 2001;80:2021–2024.

Okeson JP. Management of Temporomandibular Disorders and Occlusion. St Louis: Mosby, 2003:3–91.

Randow K, Glantz PO. On cantilever loading of vital and non-vital teeth. An experimental clinical study. Acta Odontol Scand 1986;44:271–277.

Chapter 2
Normal Function and Avoiding Damage B–F
to Restored Teeth

Aim

The aims of this chapter are to consider the importance of anterior guidance to normal function and to describe how restorations may be vulnerable to repetitive loading, especially where they are incorrectly contoured. We recommend that readers view animations B–F to bring to life the figures marked with DVD logos.

Outcome

At the end of this chapter, the clinician should:
- appreciate how teeth function during mastication
- realise that weakened and restored teeth are vulnerable to repeated stresses and strains
- understand that "guidance teeth" are important to guide the mandible to and from the intercuspal position (ICP) but will be subject to repetitive loading
- understand the terms associated with lateral excursions: *canine guidance, group function, working side* and *non-working side*, and *protrusion*
- comprehend how posterior teeth move across each other in lateral excursions
- realise the potentially catastrophic consequences of interfering with anterior guidance.

Introduction

Even in normal function, occlusal loads are repetitive and can be heavy. Although natural teeth may be able to take this load for a lifetime, teeth weakened by disease and restoration may not. Therefore, dentists need to take care to ensure that teeth are not subjected to damaging loads during normal day-to-day function. To understand how such damage may happen, it is important to understand how the teeth are involved in function. In the previous chapter, we looked at how the teeth meet in ICP, in which they transmit maximum force during eating. It is easy to appreciate how a molar weakened by a large mesio-occluso-distal restoration (or worse still, root-canal treated with incipient cracks) may suffer fracture under heavy forces developed during chewing hard foods; for example, those containing whole grains. However, even with a soft refined diet, under repeated loading teeth are at risk from excursive contacts. Understanding the nature of these contacts and how to work with them is fundamental to successful restorative dentistry.

Guidance, Natural Teeth and Function

Teeth have evolved for one major functional purpose: eating. The shape and position of the crowns and roots of teeth are no accident and have taken millions of years of evolution to acquire their current form and relationship. Practitioners, despite working on dentitions every day, sometimes forget how the masticatory system works, in particular, how harmonious function relies on teeth that guide mandibular movement into and away from ICP, providing what is termed "anterior guidance". To identify which teeth are the guidance teeth, simply ask the patient to slide their jaw out to the left or the right with the teeth in light contact and note which teeth provide "gliding" (guiding) contacts. Now repeat this with the jaw pushed forward in protrusion. It is worth remembering that the movement you are asking the patient to perform (sliding out from ICP) is the reverse of what happens during biting or chewing. It is also worth emphasising that this anterior guidance may involve both anterior and posterior teeth.

Guidance teeth are important because they come into functional contact hundreds of times each day. As such, they need to be sufficiently robust to resist the wear and tear associated with heavy and often non-axial occlusal loads.

During biting, the function of the incisors is to incise, or cut, the food in an edge-to-edge position and then guide the mandible in towards ICP along a protrusive path of excursion ("incisal guidance"). Clearly, the potential to provide such guidance will depend on the amount of overlap between the upper and lower anterior teeth. Where these teeth do not contact during protrusion, for example in a Class III incisor relationship, other teeth – canines, premolars or molars – provide the guidance.

During the chewing cycle, a bolus of food is formed and moved over the molar and premolar teeth, guided by the tongue and the cheeks. At the same time, the mandible moves laterally – often to the side with the bolus. Then the teeth crush the bolus as they close back in towards ICP, where they apply maximum force. The sequence is repeated until the bolus is eventually swallowed. As the mandible closes then opens it is guided towards and then away from ICP by the slopes of the guidance teeth. There are two main patterns of lateral excursive guidance, termed "canine guidance" and "group function" (see animations B and C on the DVD). For about half of the population, canines are the guidance teeth (Fig 2-1), having evolved for this purpose with a long and strong root to resist heavy loads. For many other people, several teeth in each arch share guidance. This group function can involve the premolars and the canines or another combination of teeth (Fig 2-2). Group function is more common in older subjects – often subsequent to the wear of the canines and tooth loss. Of course, the guidance teeth on the right may be different from those on the left, so when moving to chew on the right there might be canine guidance alone, while on the left there may be group function.

In lateral excursions, you will usually find the guidance teeth on the "working side". The working side simply means the side to which the mandible moves during a lateral excursion. Clearly, the direction of the excursion may switch from left to right during chewing. Hence, the working side is sometimes the right side and at other times the left. We define the "non-working side" as the side from which the mandible moves during a lateral excursion. Paradoxically,

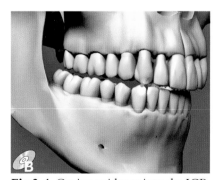

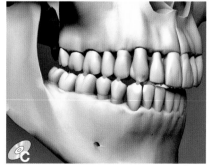

Fig 2-1 Canine guidance into the ICP. The guiding canines glide past each other while the posterior teeth remain separated until they reach ICP. This separation is called "disclusion", which occurs on both sides of the jaw in the illustration.

Fig 2-2 Another common pattern of guidance is group function, involving multiple pairs of guiding teeth.

although the term "non-working" implies that this side is not involved in chewing, this is not necessarily so. Chewing patterns vary from person to person, with many preferring to use the working side to crush the bolus. Others chew on the non-working side, bilaterally or centrally between the anterior teeth.

Tracks of Movement across Posterior Teeth

In addition to knowing which teeth guide mandibular movement, it is also important to know how the posterior teeth move across each other in excursions as this has important practical implications, particularly in terms of where you place cusps, fossae, ridges and grooves when restoring teeth so that the anatomy does not interfere with movements. The DVD illustrates relative movement of the maxillary and mandibular molars across each other. The working, non-working and protrusive movements produce distinctive tracks, what we call a "crow's foot". This is illustrated in Fig 2-3.

Guidance and Restored Teeth

Natural teeth are evolved to provide guidance and, if not subject to significant disease, can reasonably be expected to provide a lifetime of service, provided they do not wear excessively. Restored teeth are, however, inevitably weaker, and the more tooth tissue that has to be replaced, the weaker the tooth. Endontically treated teeth restored with a post-retained crown are especially vulnerable to damage during function. Such teeth have often lost more than half of their original tissue. In these situations, care with the guidance is essential when preparing for, manufacturing, and adjusting restorations. It is probably unreasonable to expect a single, heavily restored

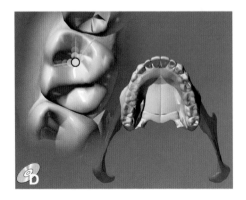

Fig 2-3 The "crow's foot" pattern of working, non-working and protrusive excursions produced by the mid-buccal cusp of the lower right first molar moving over the occlusal surface of the upper molar. The DVD will help you understand how these tracks occur across both the upper and lower teeth.

tooth to provide guidance alone. Failure to appreciate this is the cause of many failures in restorative dentistry.

There are three very simple rules to follow:
- Check the guidance on all patients before you start restoring teeth – this is very simple (see Section 8-1 for how to do this if you are unsure).
- If possible, ensure that heavily restored or vulnerable teeth are not expected to provide guidance alone. Shape the restoration to allow other teeth to take or share guidance.
- Do not change satisfactory guidance unless you are doing so to protect heavily restored or vulnerable teeth (as above).

Consequences of Interfering with Guidance

In many situations where you place crowns or large composite restorations, you will be conforming to existing guidance; in other words, you will be ensuring that the shape of the restoration duplicates the shape of the natural guidance surface it is replacing. You must undertake sufficient tooth preparation to accommodate the thickness of material, not just in the region of ICP contact, as described in Chapter 1, but also along the entire concave guiding surface. This is illustrated for a crown in Fig 2-4. As shown on the DVD (animation E), failure to remove sufficient tooth tissue in preparation will result in the guiding surface being overbulked and rather convex, with a high risk that the tooth will become overloaded by potentially damaging non-axial forces. We call such contacts "interferences". Interferences have the potential to cause problems.

A change from guidance to interference can happen quite accidentally, and with catastrophic results (Fig 2-5, DVD animation F). So what happens? In this case, as the patient uses the incisors to function or grind, the bulky palatal surface will take the entire masticatory load, repeatedly, and so something is likely to give. If it were a structurally sound tooth it may drift orthodontically, or become tender or mobile. However, this is a tooth with only a fraction of its original natural tissue left and so is likely to fail. The failure, typically where the tooth is weakest, may take various forms – the crown may fracture, the tooth may experience fatal root fracture or the restoration may debond – depending on loading and stress points. The potential for porcelain to wear opposing tooth structure is well known and is also a significant risk. Alternatively, the patient may notice that the crowned tooth becomes mobile or starts to drift out of line, in particular if the periodontal support is reduced. In other words, any weakness will be exposed.

15

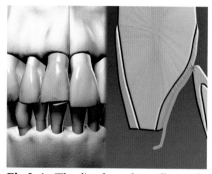

Fig 2-4a The discoloured maxillary right central incisor requires crowning. It is important to appreciate the way the palatal aspect of the incisors may be involved in guiding jaw movement; once the tooth is prepared, the guidance surface is destroyed.

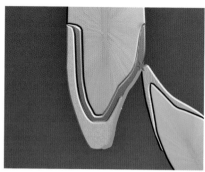

Fig 2-4b It is imperative to restore the correct guidance as well as ICP contact. The correct preparation outline provides sufficient space to accommodate the crown material (in this case a metal–ceramic crown) and, most importantly, reproduce the correct guidance.

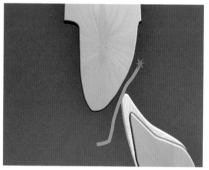

Fig 2-4c An incorrect preparation outline provides insufficient space to accommodate the crown.

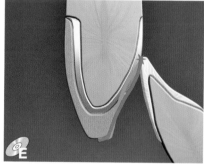

Fig 2-4d The resulting crown is bulky palatally, which can interfere with guidance (red line). This produces non-axial "jiggling" forces on the tooth, resulting in pain and other problems.

Repeatedly failing restorations should always be checked from the point of view of guidance. Crowns and post crowns are especially vulnerable to such problems, but so too are intracoronal restorations, for example composite restorations that include incisal edges. Restoration failure may happen in any part of the mouth where guidance is ignored. Simply checking and shaping

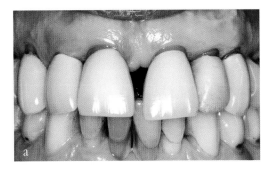
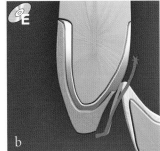
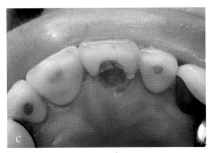
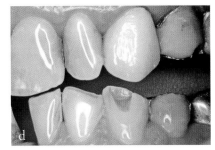

Fig 2-5 Bulky crowns have resulted in protrusive interferences causing:
(a,b) buccal displacement and production of a midline diastema – displacement and mobility are more likely to occur in teeth with reduced periodontal support;
(c) crown fracture or decementation of, in particular, post-retained crowns;
(d) wear of the opposing teeth (look at the lower left canine), especially where porcelain is left rough and unpolished after crown adjustment.

restorations to comply with the existing guidance provided by other teeth will avoid most occlusal problems. With simple plastic restorations, interferences can often be avoided by adjusting the material to ensure that guidance is re-established on the surrounding enamel.

In situations involving multiple, large composite build-ups or porcelain veneers, the restorations themselves may need to provide guidance. This requires considerable attention to detail and a mental image of the concave shape that will harmonise with mandibular movement, as well as ensuring that guidance is shared between restored teeth rather than being carried on a single restoration.

Where several teeth are being restored with crowns, it can be difficult – but all the more important – to manage guidance. There are methods to copy anterior guidance predictably into new indirect restorations. These methods are considered in Chapter 8. This is where a semi-adjustable articulator can really come into its own. The technician can simulate the jaw movements and shape the restorations to give you whatever guidance is most appropriate for the patient.

So far, we have focused on normal function, ICP and guidance teeth, and what may happen if you change tooth contacts to interfere with guidance. We will consider further the concepts of interferences and deflective contacts in Chapter 3, and in particular what happens when the cusps of the posterior teeth interfere with excursive movement or deflect mandibular movement. We will also examine the problems caused to teeth and restorations by parafunction.

Conclusions

- Restored teeth are at greater risk than intact teeth from repeated masticatory loading.
- Practitioners need to know how tooth movements are influenced by mandibular excursions.
- Before restoring a tooth, the practitioner needs to check if it is involved in guidance.
- If it is, guidance harmonious with mandibular movement should be re-established when the restoration is placed.
- During tooth preparation, ensure there is sufficient space to accommodate the restoration without interfering with excursive movements.
- Be vigilant in observing clinical problems associated with interferences.

Further Reading

Ash MM, Nelson SJ. Wheeler's Dental Anatomy, Physiology, and Occlusion. Philadelphia: Saunders, 2003.

Klineberg I, Jagger R. Occlusion and Clinical Practice: an Evidence-based Approach. Edinburgh: Wright, 2004.

Chapter 3
Deflective Contacts, Interferences G–I and Parafunction

Aim

The aim of this chapter is to emphasise the importance of deflective contacts, interferences and parafunction in causing damage to both teeth and restorations. We recommend that readers view animations G–I to bring to life figures marked with DVD logos.

Outcome

At the end of this chapter, the clinician should:
- understand what is meant by the terms *centric relation (CR)*, *retruded contact position* (RCP) and *slide between RCP and intercuspal position (ICP)*
- recognise the influence of damaging *deflective contacts*, *anterior thrust* and *interferences*
- realise the potential consequences of tooth preparation on "pivoting" deflective and interfering contacts
- understand what is meant by *parafunction* and the damage it may cause
- realise that if problems of occlusal overloading (unexplained pain, attrition, *abfraction*, drifting and mobility, as well as damage and decementation of restorations) are not explained by function they may be explained by parafunction.

Introduction

In Chapter 2 we talked about normal, functional movements of the mandible, where guidance teeth take on the role of smoothly directing the movement of the mandible into the ICP. We also introduced the concept of interferences to that smooth movement: tooth contacts that disrupt movement by getting in the way. In the first half of this chapter, we introduce the concept of deflective contacts and further explore the potentially deleterious properties of interferences. In the second half, we consider parafunction and the ways in which its effects can be especially damaging to teeth, restorations and supporting tissues.

Deflective Contacts and Excursive Interferences

So far, we have built our understanding of occlusion using ICP as a starting point. This position is fundamentally important to occlusion, but it is dictated entirely by the teeth. To understand interferences and deflective contacts fully we need to take on board the concept of CR, a concept that is not at all related to the teeth, but is completely dictated by the temporomandibular joints (TMJs).

Centric Relation

During function, the mandible travels towards ICP within an envelope of movement defined by the guidance surfaces of the anterior teeth. So far, we have considered the lateral and protrusive guiding surfaces, but at least 90% of the population are also able to move their jaws distal to ICP. This is because for most of us there is a small discrepancy between the musculoskeletally stable position of the mandible, which is determined by the TMJs, and the position of stability determined by the teeth (ICP).

The stable position of the condyles within the TMJs is known as CR. This is defined variously as the most superior-posterior, most superior or most superior-anterior position of the condyles within the glenoid fossae (see Fig 3-1). While academics continue to argue about which of these positions they are talking about, this argument is of little practical relevance. Dentists take a more pragmatic approach to find CR and use manipulative techniques, which comfortably seat the condyles into their most superior position within the glenoid fossae. In this position, the articular discs should be correctly interposed and the mandible can arc around its "terminal hinge axis". It is a position of

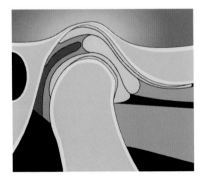

Fig 3-1 CR with the condyles in their most superior position in the glenoid fossae with the discs correctly interposed.

Yellow – fibrocartilage disc and joint surfaces; *light brown* – superior and inferior lateral pterygoid muscles; *dark brown* – vascular retrodiscal tissues; *green* – superior and inferior retrodiscal laminae; *blue* – synovial fluid in superior and inferior joint spaces.

health that does not occur in a diseased TMJ in which, for example, there is a disc displacement or arthritis. To find CR we use the technique of bimanual manipulation to guide the mandible; this is such an important and useful skill for understanding occlusion that there is an entire section in this book (Section 8-4) and DVD video (M) to explain how to do it.

Retruded Contact Position

This is simply the relationship between the mandible and maxilla on the terminal hinge axis when the first point of tooth contact occurs. This usually occurs between the posterior teeth (see Fig 3-2). From here the mandible can slide into ICP. The DVD animation G shows this clearly. In a proportion of the population (usually around 10%) this point of contact is ICP; in other words, the patient hinges straight into ICP because ICP lies on that retruded arc of closure. In the remaining 90% of the population there is a slide from the RCP into ICP.

RCP–ICP Slide

This slide is usually 0.5 to 1 mm in length when viewed at the incisors, but depending on the nature of the tooth contact it can be up to several millimetres long. The direction of the slide is best described in terms of vertical, horizontal and lateral components (see Figs 3-3 and 3-4). To assess a slide you need to view what happens at the incisors from both the side and the front of the patient. With a vertical slide, the mandible moves little, if any, from its retruded arc of closure. With a horizontal slide, the mandible translates forwards so that the lower incisors appear to move both upwards and anteriorly when viewed from

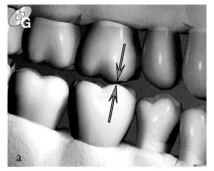
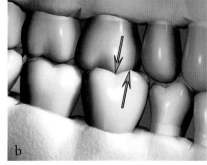

Fig 3-2 (a) RCP: the first tooth contact in CR; (b) the mandible then slides into ICP.

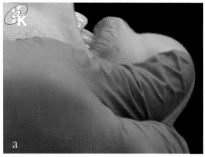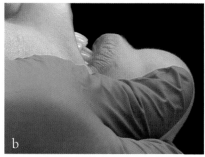

Fig 3-3 Bimanual manipulation of the RCP–ICP slide viewed laterally. (a) Incisor relationship in RCP. (b) Incisor relationship in ICP – the mandible has moved superiorly and anteriorly to this position. The forwards translation (here about 1.5 mm) is the horizontal component of the slide.

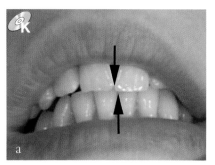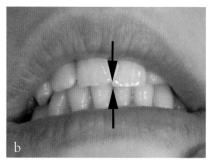

Fig 3-4 The same slide from RCP–ICP as Fig 3-3 viewed anteriorly. (a) Incisors separated by posterior RCP contact between the upper and lower left second premolars. (b) Incisor relationship in ICP. Arrows show the lateral component of the slide.

the side. With a lateral slide the mandible rotates slightly, with one condyle moving further forward in the slide than the other does. The result is that the mandibular incisor midline shows a shift either to the right or the left between RCP and ICP (see Fig 3-4). The patient examined before an occlusal adjustment in DVD video K (see Sections 8-1 and 8-7) illustrates both horizontal and lateral components of slide.

Deflective Contact

This is a tooth contact that deflects the mandible from one path of closure to another. As the RCP–ICP slide deflects the mandible into ICP, we consider the tooth contacts involved as deflective contacts. If the slide is removed by grinding away the deflective contacts, most patients will function back to RCP. These deflective contacts are often involved during function when a person chews towards the side where the contact occurs, creating a telltale wear facet on the affected teeth. Some deflective contacts can be damaging, the simplest example being an overerupting maxillary third molar deflecting against the distal aspect of a lower second molar (DVD animation G). Invariably, occlusal instability leading to unwanted tooth movements gives rise to damaging and uncomfortable deflective contacts (Fig 3-5). Sometimes these contacts are large and obvious, but at other times they are surprisingly small. What is surprising is that apparently similar deflective contacts produce markedly different reactions; one patient may be totally unaware of its existence but another may have problems, such as pain in and around the tooth, often associated with bruxism. In terms of patient presentation, it is perhaps not so much the contact but the patient's reaction to it that is important. We consider the relationship of deflective contacts to bruxism at the end of this chapter.

Anterior Thrust

Although the teeth directly involved in the RCP–ICP slide can show signs of wear (faceting) and heavy occlusal contact (vertical enamel fracture lines), the damage caused by the slide may lie elsewhere. Classically, the slide causes an "anterior thrust" of the mandible during function or parafunction, resulting in the mandibular incisors impinging heavily onto the palatal surfaces of the maxillary incisors. The resulting non-axial loading can, in turn, cause or accelerate localised wear, typically with drifting and mobility – usually of the maxillary incisors. Of course, periodontal disease (see Chapter 5) also causes drifting and mobility of anterior teeth and needs to be treated, but its resolution

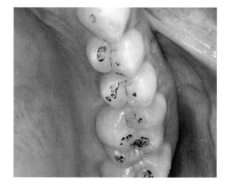

Fig 3-5 Occlusal instability indicated by broad rubbing contacts and associated history of occlusal changes and functional disturbance.

23

may be dependent on removal of an anterior thrust through occlusal adjustment or splint treatment. As a rule, when problems occur with anterior teeth that involve wear, drifting, mobility and atypical loss of bone support, it is always wise, and easy, to check the posterior teeth for deflective contacts.

Excursive Interferences

In Chapter 2 we considered how a poorly contoured crown acts as a protrusive interference. Interferences are contacts on a tooth or restoration that interfere with smooth mandibular excursive movements. Like deflective contacts, they are sometimes associated with bruxism; they possibly act as a trigger, but more likely cause problems by adversely affecting the distribution of heavy occlusal forces. Again, occlusal adjustment or splint treatment may be helpful to harmonise mandibular movement.

Pivoting Contacts

Both interferences and deflective contacts can act as pivots, causing the mandible to rock around the pivot point. This in turn causes either the separation of teeth anterior to the pivot or the distraction of one or both of the condyles. Pivot contacts can cause problems during preparation for restorations including crowns and onlays.

Sometimes, interocclusal space seems mysteriously to disappear during or soon after crown preparation, despite allowing sufficient reduction to give adequate occlusal clearance. The disappearance of 1–2 mm of clearance in such a short time is clearly not a consequence of overeruption. A more likely explanation for this problem is the effects of altering occlusal pivots; the "last tooth in the arch syndrome" is the classical example. This is a bit difficult to grasp sometimes, but Fig 3-6 and DVD animation H show how it works.

Interferences on the working side can act as anteroposterior pivots too (Fig 3-7), while non-working-side interferences can act as cross-arch pivots (Fig 3-8 and DVD animation I). Again, removal of these pivots during crown preparation can result in loss of interocclusal space.

The first step in dealing with this problem is to know it exists prior to tooth preparation. As described in Chapter 2, knowing which are the guidance teeth is an essential starting point. Any disruption to guidance can be followed up by looking for interferences causing significant deflective contacts, while manipulating the patient into the retruded hinge axis.

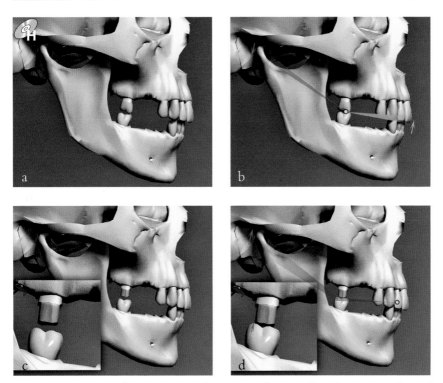

Fig 3-6 Pivoting deflective contact between right second molars causing loss of occlusal space following crown preparation.
(a) Teeth in RCP. (b) Teeth in ICP with condylar distraction around pivot. (c) Pivot removed during crown preparation. (d) Condyle positions superiorly with loss of interocclusal space.

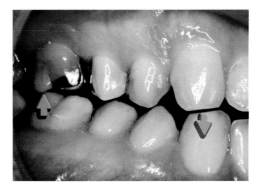

Fig 3-7 Anteroposterior pivot caused by a working-side interference between the first molars in right lateral excursion. Notice how the pivot lifts the faceted canines out of occlusion.

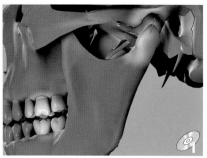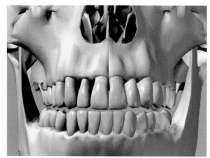

Fig 3-8 Cross-arch pivot caused by a non-working-side interference against the upper left first molar in right lateral excursion, viewed laterally and anteriorly. Notice how the pivot lifts the canines on the right side out of contact and distracts the condyle on the left side away from its fossa.

Should a pivoting contact be detected on a tooth to be crowned or onlayed, the strategies for dealing with it are:

- Simply prepare the crown and anticipate a greater occlusal reduction than normal. Once sufficient reduction has been achieved it is generally wise to fit a provisional restoration and delay recording the impression and jaw registration until the following appointment. Should there be any alteration in jaw position in the interim, this can be compensated for by means of further occlusal reduction.
- Carry out an occlusal adjustment at an appointment prior to preparation to eliminate the pivot. Should the pivot be a deflective contact, adjusting it will move the retruded contact onto another pair of teeth. This may be all you need to do, but you may consider a more comprehensive approach (see Chapter 8).
- In cases in which the patient is symptomless and the pivoting contact is very large, occlusal adjustment may cause excessive dentine exposure. This situation is rare, but when it occurs the reduction and associated preparation may need to be completed with due regard to the sufficiency of the remaining dentine thickness. Dentists sometimes try and copy the pivoting contact into the new restoration, but this is notoriously difficult.

Parafunction and Its Problems

Sound teeth cope well with normal function, but not with abnormal function. The term "parafunction" is used to include a range of abnormal habits or actions, including clenching, grinding (bruxism) and tongue thrusting. Parafunction, in particular bruxism, can be very damaging to sound and restored teeth alike.

Bruxism is defined as a movement disorder of the masticatory system that is characterised, among other things, by teeth grinding and clenching, during sleep as well as wakefulness. The large forces produced during bruxism can have detrimental effects on dental, periodontal and musculoskeletal tissues. The problems associated with bruxism are many and varied. The dental problems include unexplained dental pain, increased tooth wear caused by attrition (Fig 3-9) and abfraction (Fig 3-10).

When teeth are weakened by restoration and have to cope with parafunctional loading, the result can be rapid and catastrophic restoration failure, including wear leading to restoration perforation (Fig 3-11) or decementation and fracture of the restored tooth unit. Problems often include drifting, mobility and, in susceptible patients, an accelerated rate of bone loss associated with periodontal disease (see Chapter 5). Musculoskeletal problems are also more likely to occur, sometimes producing signs and symptoms of temporomandibular disorder (TMD) (see Chapter 7).

Fig 3-9 Generalised wear, worse on anterior teeth, associated with protrusive bruxism. The patient bruxed during the day and, according to his wife, at night also. Notice the vertical enamel cracks in the maxillary central incisors, indicative of heavy occlusal loading.

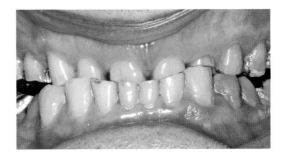

Fig 3-10 Abfraction lesions; V-shaped cervical notches caused, at least in part, by stress corrosion resulting from heavy parafunctional loading in excursions. Abfraction is often difficult to differentiate from non-carious cervical tooth substance loss of other aetiology.

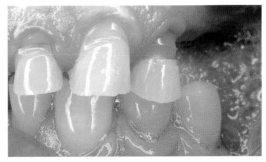

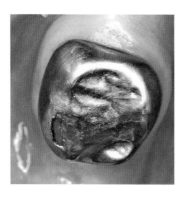

Fig 3-11 Worn and perforated crown in a bruxist.

Parafunction, in particular bruxism, can be extremely damaging to restorations. As a consequence, providing complex and expensive restorations for bruxists can be a soul-destroying experience, as they are likely to fail. The chapters on occlusal reorganisation, periodontal disease, implants and TMD contain repeated references to the risks when treating bruxists. There are also questions about the role of occlusion in parafunction, and whether careful occlusal management will reduce loading, or at least rearrange the occlusal contacts, in such a way as to limit damaging effects.

Aetiology of Bruxism

The reason we have included bruxism here is that, rather like TMD, the aetiology of bruxism was for many years thought to be entirely due to occlusal discrepancies, including deflective contacts and interferences. This is sometimes the case, but there is now considerable evidence to show that nocturnal bruxism is centrally mediated, involving sleep arousal and disturbances in the dopaminergic system. Underlying these disturbances may be psychosocial factors. In other words, it can be influenced by normal day-to-day "stress" manifesting at night, and there is a possible genetic susceptibility. Certain commonly prescribed drugs, such as SSRIs (selective serotonin re-uptake inhibitors), cause some patients to brux, as does the use of some recreational drugs, for example amphetamines. Some neurological or psychiatric diseases also have bruxism as a feature.

Occlusal discrepancies such as deflective contacts and interferences can have a role in aetiology of bruxism, but appear to be more strongly associated with daytime, rather than night-time, parafunction. Patients are often aware that they grind on a certain tooth or teeth, and, as described earlier in this chapter,

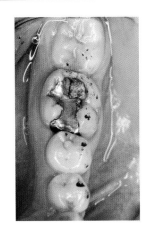

Fig 3-12 Restoration breakdown associated with bruxism on non-working-side interference (marked in red; ICP contacts marked in black).

this can be irritating for the patient. Sometimes placement of an interfering restoration coincides with the start of a grinding habit. The classic example is when, following placement of an amalgam restoration, a patient reports pain and a "squeaking" occlusal contact. Clinically, there appears a telltale, shiny facet and signs of occlusal overload, indicating that the patient has been grinding on this spot (Fig 3-12). Another common scenario occurs after fitting a crown or veneer in which the premature contact or interference causing discomfort may be close to ICP, or along what should have been the guidance surface. If you see a problem unexplained by normal function, consider parafunction.

Management of Bruxism

In the past, dentists held deflective contacts and interferences largely responsible for triggering bruxism. Such occlusal discrepancies usually cause no clinical problems and it would be foolish to remove them indiscriminately as a preventive measure. In other situations, the patient cannot find a comfortable position in which to close the teeth and, like scratching an itch, bruxes against the deflective contact or contacts (Fig 3-5). It is difficult to be certain whether such contacts are a cause or a result of bruxism, but their removal does seem to provide comfort for some patients who grind during the day rather than just at night. This approach does not work in all cases. For nocturnal bruxism an occlusal stabilisation splint (see Section 8-10) is the preferred treatment. Such splints work by providing occlusal stability around CR and preventing direct tooth-to-tooth contact. In some patients the parafunctional activity is reduced, but not in others with an ingrained habit. The evidence for bruxism is simple to find clinically using a splint: look for marked wear facets on, or perforation

29

of, the splint's occlusal surface. The splint will, however, protect the teeth from further wear. The flat surface limits the effects of the heavy and potentially damaging occlusal forces, which would otherwise be directed on to the deflective contacts and interferences.

Conclusions

- CR is a reproducible musculoskeletal position that needs to be considered as part of an occlusal examination.
- Deflective contacts between RCP and ICP are usually innocuous but can produce occlusal problems and discomfort, in particular in cases in which the occlusion is unstable and the patient is a bruxist.
- Deflective contacts and interferences sometimes act as pivots. Following their removal during tooth preparation, a loss of interocclusal space can occur. Pivots need to be identified and managed appropriately.
- The heavy forces produced during bruxism can have detrimental effects on dental, periodontal and musculoskeletal tissues.
- Nocturnal bruxism is centrally mediated rather than occlusally mediated.
- Dental management of nocturnal bruxism usually involves splint treatment, together with occlusal adjustment, which is sometimes helpful to redistribute loading.

Further Reading

Attanasio R. An overview of bruxism and its management. Dent Clin North Am 1997;41(2):229–241.

Lobbezoo F, Naeije M. Bruxism is mainly regulated centrally, not peripherally. J Oral Rehabil 2001;28(12):1085–1091.

Lobbezoo F, Van Der Zaag J, Naeije M. Bruxism: its multiple causes and its effects on dental implants – an updated review. J Oral Rehabil 2006;33(4):293–300.

Lyons K. Aetiology of abfraction lesions. N Z Dent J 2001;97(429):93–98.

Manfredini D, Cantini E, Romagnoli M, Bosco M. Prevalence of bruxism in patients with different research diagnostic criteria for temporomandibular disorders (RDC/TMD) diagnoses. Cranio 2003;21(4):279–285.

Okeson JP. Orofacial Pain. Guidelines for Assessment, Diagnosis and Management Chicago: Quintessence, 1996.

Chapter 4
Reorganising the Occlusion

Aim

The aim of this chapter is to demystify "reorganising the occlusion" so as to make this important aspect of dental care more accessible, but at the same time to highlight potential areas of difficulty.

Outcome

At the end of this chapter, the clinician should:
- understand the difference between reorganising an occlusion and conforming with the presenting intercuspal position (ICP)
- recognise when occlusal reorganisation is indicated
- be familiar with the principles involved in occlusal reorganisation:
  - using centric relation (CR) as the starting point for reconstruction
  - deciding on the vertical dimension
  - designing the pattern of occlusal contacts in ICP and mandibular excursions
- appreciate the practicalities of reorganising, including the recognition of cases that are potentially more difficult.

Introduction

A "reorganised occlusion" is an occlusion in which the pattern of occlusal contacts is deliberately changed or reconstructed.

Reorganising the occlusion is not something that needs to be undertaken for many patients, but there are times when such action is the only way, let alone the most appropriate and easiest means, to solve a clinical problem. It is a procedure that has to be done with care. Its exponents often make it appear mystical or impossibly technical. Actually, the underlying principles are very simple and will be familiar to all practitioners. Occlusal reorganisation should not, therefore, be viewed as intimidating. That said, the importance of the basic technicalities should not be underestimated, and careful thought and preparation are needed prior to the application of the technical skills necessary to complete the procedure successfully.

One of the reasons that this can seem a deeply intimidating subject is that reorganising the occlusion cannot simply be done by following an instruction manual. Every case is different, reflecting the huge diversity of form and condition of teeth and their relationships. Consequently, it is essential to grasp the principles fully before thinking through the technical detail for any given individual.

In a sense, reorganising the occlusion brings together all of the basic occlusal concepts that were introduced in Chapters 1 to 3. In this chapter, we will refer back to these chapters, and their animations, and forwards to Chapter 8, along with its videos detailing clinical procedures.

Why Bother?

The answer to this is relatively simple. You reorganise an occlusion because the existing ICP is unsatisfactory for your restorations, or because there is a specific problem that really can only be solved by reorganising the occlusion. That is all very well, but it is still not very clear which clinical circumstances dictate or suggest reorganisation. This question is perhaps best answered with some examples. Those given below are not the only circumstances where you may wish to reorganise, but they do illustrate a range of situations where reorganising may either be necessary or worth the effort and cost. Decisions about whether to conform to an existing occlusion or to reorganise it are not always black and white.

Example 1: The Complete Denture

Making a complete denture may not seem like reorganising the occlusion, but that is exactly what it is. The complete denture has an occlusion that is built from nothing. If there are no teeth, there can be no occlusion (Fig 4-1). Whenever you make a new set of complete dentures, you effectively have to rebuild the occlusion such that the teeth fit together without displacing the denture every time the mouth is closed. This rebuilt occlusion is, to a greater or lesser degree, reorganised, even if you try to recreate what was there before. Normally, though, you start afresh, using as your starting point a jaw position determined by the temporomandibular joints (TMJs), which is of course CR, as described in the previous chapter (Fig 3-1).

Although making dentures may not seem to fit a common image of reorganising the occlusion, the basic principles used to make complete dentures are the same as those used to reorganise the occlusion for dentate people. However, as

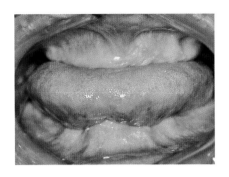

Fig 4-1 "Big Mac": where there are no teeth there is no ICP. Instead, the TMJs are used as the starting point for denture construction, with the occlusion reorganised around CR.

we will see, although CR is used as the starting point to create a new ICP for both complete dentures and natural teeth, there are significant differences in the way the excursive contacts are arranged. With complete dentures, the widely accepted ideal is to have bilateral excursive contacts occurring simultaneously between as many anterior and posterior teeth as possible. This "balanced articulation" is simply the means to stop the dentures from tipping during function. Balanced articulation is an example of an "occlusal scheme", and selecting an occlusal scheme is an important part of reorganising. We discuss occlusal schemes later in the chapter, but Box 4-1 gives a flavour of their history.

Box 4-1 **Balanced articulation**

Balanced articulation has long been used to construct complete dentures, but it does not perform well when used to reconstruct dentate patients – as both the Gnathologists and Pankey–Mann–Schuyler groups discovered to their embarrassment in the middle of the 20th century. These two groups of dentists, working independently on the west and east coasts of America, did much to pioneer the practicalities of occlusal reconstruction. Each group had its own characteristic techniques and instrumentation. For almost 30 years both groups restored dentate patients with balanced articulations. Then, in the late 1950s, both groups acknowledged that there were problems with this approach: patients often suffered discomfort from heavy non-working-side contacts. Furthermore, these interferences appeared to cause wear, fracture and mobility of the restored teeth. Consequently, for dentate patients both groups abandoned balanced articulation in favour of what they observed to work naturally in healthy dentitions. The Gnathologists favoured canine guidance while the Pankey–Mann–Schuyler followers preferred group function, but both stipulated disclusion of the posterior teeth on the non-working side and in protrusion (see Table 4-1).

Table 4-1 **Features of some of the best known occlusal schemes** (Derived from Wassell RW, Steele JG, Welsh G. Considerations when planning occlusal rehabilitation: a review of the literature. Int Dent J 1998;48:571–581)

Occlusal scheme	RCP–ICP relationship	Excursive contacts	Comments
Gnathological (1964)	Coincident, with tripod contacts	Canine-guided lateral excursions, posterior disclusion in all excursions. Anterior and posterior contacts are mutually protected[1]	Good for restoring cases without a large horizontal component of RCP–ICP slide. Real purists would insist on the use of a fully adjustable articulator and all that goes with it.
Youdelis (1977)	Coincident, with tripod contacts	As for gnathological, but designed to drop into group function if canines wear or move	Useful option where excursive parafunction cannot be controlled or where the canine is compromised
Pankey–Mann–Schuyler (1963)	Area of freedom[2] between ICP and RCP (<0.5 mm) and morphology functionally generated	Anterior guidance determined functionally on temporaries. Either canine guided or group function	The potential for error with the functionally generated path technique, which is used to determine the occlusal morphology of posterior teeth is considerable
Area of freedom in centric (1982)	Area of freedom between ICP and RCP (0.5 mm ± 0.3 mm); cusp to fossa occlusion	Either canine guided or group function, but anterior guidance will be delayed during posterior contact in area of freedom	Useful where there has been a large horizontal component in the RCP–ICP slide before treatment. Area of freedom needs careful adjustment

Table 4–1 **Features of some of the best known occlusal schemes** (continued)

Occlusal scheme	RCP–ICP relationship	Excursive contacts	Comments
Balanced occlusion (1960)	Area of freedom between ICP and RCP	Balanced working and non–working contacts in lateral excursions. Balanced anterior and posterior contacts in occlusion	Keeps complete dentures stable during excursions, but difficult to manage in the natural dentition and risk of non–working–side overloading
Nyman and Lindhe (1983)	RCP and ICP must have even contact	Bilaterally balanced excursive contacts determined in provisional (long–term temporary) restorations and then copied into definitive restorations	This is used in cross arch bridges where there is advanced, but controlled, periodontal disease. Balanced contacts give stability to an otherwise mobile bridge

Notes:

1: "Mutually protected" means that in ICP the posterior teeth support maximum biting force while the anterior teeth are just out of contact, but in excursions the anterior teeth provide guidance to disclude the posterior teeth and protect them from lateral loading. To avoid locking the condyles into CR, this guidance should start shallow and then become steeper.

2: Area of freedom (freedom in centric) is designed to prevent condyles being locked into CR.

Example 2: Rebuilding the Aging Dentition

In a mouth affected by decades of dental disease there is often extensive tooth loss and multiple restorations. This is now a common occurrence in people from late middle age onwards. The result, after years of repeated cycles of damage and restoration, is a patchwork of spaces and heavily restored teeth. Remaining teeth drift and overerupt, and many may have huge restorations or poorly constructed crowns. An example of this sort of problem is shown in Fig 4-2. There comes a point where a path has to be chosen: the dentist and the patient have to make a decision. Do you leave things ticking over and patched up to conform to what is there, or will this lead to difficult problems in the future? Does a bold step need to be made to remove the remaining teeth and reorganise the occlusion with a complete denture or implant-retained prosthesis? Or, would it be better to use the remaining natural teeth as a basis for building a stable, functional and aesthetic (reorganised) occlusion, and if so is it a sensible investment? The application of basic principles is important, and some lateral thought and imagination may be required to do this successfully.

Example 3: Protecting and Restoring a Worn Dentition

When teeth suffer excessive wear this can affect appearance and function, as well as causing symptoms of sensitivity and pulp damage. The reasons for wear are discussed elsewhere and, clearly, understanding why it has occurred is important in planning its management. Irrespective of cause, if treatment is indicated to make the teeth look better, to prevent the symptoms associated

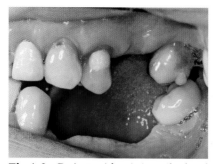

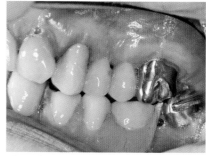

Fig 4-2a Patient with missing, tilted and heavily restored teeth. Before reconstruction, deflective contacts and interferences were removed.

Fig 4-2b Notice the lower occlusal plane levelled with a new gold crown to eliminate the presenting protrusive interference.

with wear or to prevent the wear progressing, the teeth need to be covered or reconstructed with some sort of restorative material. The extent of treatment will depend on whether wear is localised or generalised and how heavily restored the teeth are.

You can manage localised wear of anterior teeth quite simply by making space for restorative material through building up selected teeth using a Dahl approach (Fig 4-3). This results in adaptive occlusal changes, including the posterior teeth "erupting" back into contact. This approach is considered in detail in Section 8-11.

If the wear is more widespread, or the posterior teeth require extracoronal restorations, then a more extensive plan is needed. More teeth (sometimes all teeth) need to be covered or rebuilt so that the upper and lower teeth fit together again in a stable scheme that spreads the occlusal load predictably around the dental arches. This is classically what we think of as reorganising the occlusion. It may even include teeth not worn in the first place to develop an appropriate occlusal scheme. A case undertaken following the application

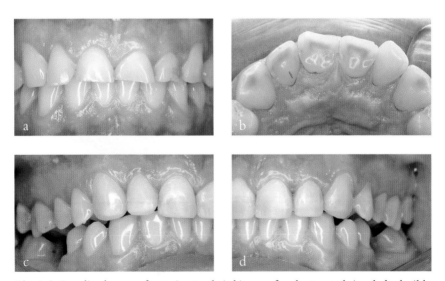

Fig 4-3 Localised wear of anterior teeth (a,b) can often be treated simply by building up the worn teeth (c,d) to allow adaptive occlusal changes (Dahl concept), by means of direct composites. Posterior occlusal contact will be re-established after several months.

of the basic principles is shown in Fig 4-4. The reconstruction of an extensive wear case complicated by an active and damaging parafunctional habit is shown in Fig 4-5. It has now been in place for over 20 years.

Example 4: Reorganising a Traumatic Occlusion

Sometimes the existing occlusion can become destructive to itself through naturally developing occlusal discrepancies or, more commonly, through dentists placing occlusally defective restorations (Fig 4-6). For example, in Chapter 3 we described how a large discrepancy between CR and ICP (an RCP–ICP slide) can result in localised damage to teeth, restorations, periodontium and, occasionally, the masticatory muscles and TMJs. The patient featured in the DVD had developed this type of functional problem associated with a lateral component to the RCP–ICP slide (see Chapter 8), causing her to be highly aware of her teeth being misaligned and uncomfortable.

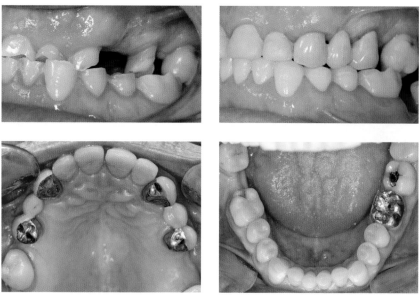

Fig 4-4 A case of generalised wear. Anterior composite build-ups increased the vertical dimension. Having created space posteriorly, a combination of bridgework and direct occlusal composites were used to stabilise the occlusion. The future strategy is to replace any rapidly failing composites with crowns, using crown lengthening where necessary to ensure an adequate ferrule on sound tooth tissue.

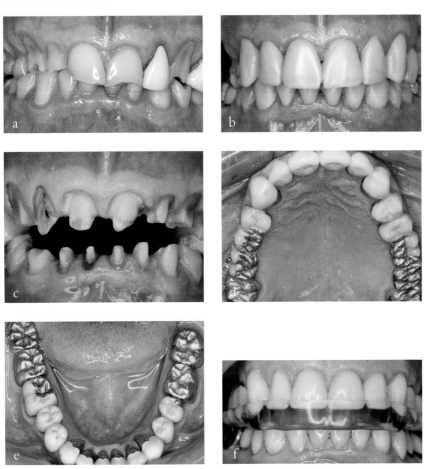

Fig 4-5 Reorganisation at increased vertical dimension.
(a) The patient had erosive and attritive wear with associated bruxism. (b) The vertical dimension was increased on anterior provisional restorations, with interim posterior stability being provided using composite directly bonded to the occlusal surfaces of the molars and premolars. (c) Tooth preparations anteriorly. Note how destructive preparations are to lower incisors – where possible, try and avoid crown preparations on such teeth. (d,e) Occlusal views showing choice of material to prevent differential wear: porcelain against porcelain and metal against metal. (f) A stabilisation splint, fitted following treatment to protect, in particular, the porcelain from damage.

It might appear both sensible and possible to remove the cause of the damage by immediately adjusting or reshaping the teeth, starting with the damaging contact. However, an unstable CR may complicate attempts to achieve

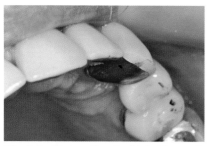

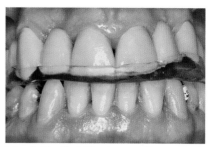

Fig 4-6a Patient fitted with bridgework covering most of the upper arch but with defective occlusion causing pain and Grade III mobility of the upper left canine abutment.

Fig 4-6b Stabilisation appliance fitted and adjusted over eight appointments before the occlusion became stable and the patient comfortable. Occlusal adjustment was then performed and the bridge replaced, taking care to provide occlusal stability and correct guidance.

occlusal stability, necessitating a period of initial splint therapy before irreversibly equilibrating and restoring the teeth. This problem is illustrated in Fig 4-6. If in doubt, it is advisable first to establish stability on a splint, as described in Section 8-10. Furthermore, unless the adjustment is obvious and simple, it needs to be carefully planned with the aid of mounted casts, as described in Section 8-8.

These four examples are far from exhaustive. Many cases will involve elements of two or more of them. We could probably fill a book with scenarios, each with several possible solutions, but there still may not be one that matches the next occlusal problem you encounter. Solving such problems often involves ingenuity, and that can only happen if the basic principles are understood. Let us now consider these principles.

The Principles of Reorganising G M

Principle 1: Rebuild the New Occlusion around a Reproducible Position
In situations in which there are no teeth, or the existing ICP is unsatisfactory, CR is normally used as the basis for reconstructing a new ICP. With the condyles fully seated in CR, the mandible will rotate open and closed around an arc that is reproducible, like a hinge. This is covered in detail in Chapter 3, but it may be worth looking at DVD animation G again by way of a reminder. If you can consistently manage to get your patient into this hinge

axis, everything else that follows becomes easier. If you want to learn how to do this, go to Section 8-4; DVD video M shows it demonstrated. Undoubtedly, manipulating a patient's mandible in this way is an acquired skill, which improves with practice. If you practise it on every new patient, it becomes easy for the vast majority of patients. A few patients can, however, cause problems, even for experienced operators.

If you cannot effectively manipulate your patient in CR, it is best not to embark on reorganising the occlusion. The problem may simply be down to your technique, but there are two other potential reasons. First, it may be because the patient is inherently difficult to manipulate. In Section 8-4 we consider methods of overcoming a patient's subconscious, but stubborn, tendency to arc only into ICP, or even into protrusion. Second, there may be an underlying temporomandibular disorder (TMD). If the patient has a TMD, the general principle is first to diagnose it (see Chapter 7) and then treat it by conservative means before embarking on restorative work. It is unwise to encourage your patient to expect a reorganised occlusion to cure their TMD.

Principle 2: Decide on the Vertical Dimension

Building the occlusion "somewhere" on that CR hinge axis is all very well, but a decision needs to be made where to stop on the arc. In other words, at what vertical height will the occlusion be reorganised? When making a complete denture, it is the rest position that is used as a reference point, with dentures usually registered a few millimetres further closed. When teeth are present, the rules change. In fact, there are no fixed rules, as the rest position readjusts to accommodate most reasonable increases in vertical dimension, as long as a stable occlusal scheme is provided.

If you need to increase the vertical dimension to construct aesthetic restorations, then the amount of space needed for your restorations will usually determine the new vertical dimension. With worn teeth, it may be the amount by which the anterior teeth need to be lengthened to make them look reasonable (Figs 4-4 and 4-5), or in a broken-down partial dentition it may be the increase necessary to obtain a level occlusal plane. An increase in the vertical dimension in the former is usually essential; in the latter it is often invaluable. Decisions about the space required are usually best made utilising a diagnostic wax-up (see Section 8-8). It is not sensible to increase the vertical dimension more than is really necessary, but the capacity of the neuromuscular system to adapt is considerable. Often, where teeth have lost height through wear, or where there is "overclosure" as a result of tooth loss or drifting, several millimetres of opening may be well tolerated. Measuring the freeway space might give an indication as to whether the wear has been compensated by continued dentoalveolar growth – in which case the freeway space will be a normal 2–3 mm, but such measurements are not particularly reliable.

Traditionally, a stabilisation splint would have been recommended to test any change in vertical dimension prior to placing expensive fixed restorations. With the use of adhesive techniques, such as composite build-ups, a splint is not a prerequisite. In the experience of the authors, problems of intolerance are rare, in particular in cases in which only a few millimetres are required. However, an occlusal stabilisation splint is often a good way of supporting the occlusion while restorations are placed (see Section 8-12 for strategies used to increase the vertical dimension). Where new restorations are at risk of damage from parafunction, a stabilisation splint is essential for protection. In such cases it is helpful to know that the patient can tolerate a splint before embarking on extensive treatment.

Principle 3: Create Stability in ICP and Avoid Damage in Excursions – You Need an Occlusal Scheme

Various occlusal schemes are described in the literature. We have already described balanced articulation as an occlusal scheme for dentures, but, as set out in Table 4-1, other schemes are available for various applications. This quick review reveals that all schemes use CR as the starting point for construction, but there is an array of subtle differences in the choice of guidance teeth and the pattern of ICP contacts. The truth is that all of these schemes are based on theory or on observations of what seems to work; none is backed up by really meaningful scientific evidence. All of the schemes are designed to optimise the transmission of occlusal forces while providing stability and harmony to allow the patient to adapt.

The small differences between schemes are usually not very important. The most important thing is to have a predetermined plan as to how your patient's teeth will fit together and which teeth will provide guidance – in other words, you should have thought about it before you start. The worst occlusal scheme is the arbitrary occlusal scheme, which may inadvertently build in damaging premature contacts, deflective contacts and interferences.

The New ICP

The ICP is usually quite stable, with the maxillary and mandibular teeth fitting together like a lock and key. When a new ICP is built, this needs to be stable too. In other words, cusps and fossae need to fit together securely when the jaws are closed. If they do not then there is a risk of drift, overeruption or damage, as described in Chapter 1.

The concept of an "ideal occlusion" may be used as a starting point for designing an occlusal scheme reorganised with extensive extracoronal restorations. Indeed, most of the animations on the DVD are built around something approaching an ideal occlusion. The concept of an ideal occlusion is fine as a starting point, but has to be adapted to the real world.

Occlusal surfaces will be stable provided that cusps and preferably fossae, rather than the marginal ridges of opposing teeth, are aligned to direct loads down long axes rather than obliquely (Fig 1-7). Traditionally, where multiple fixed restorations are being provided, a cusp to fossa arrangement would be considered more stable and less likely to cause problems – for example, food packing – than an arrangement where the cusps occlude on opposing marginal ridges, as they often do in nature. Like so much in dentistry, these ideals are not supported by meaningful evidence, but they at least give a technician something to aim for. The gnathological literature goes further, demanding that the perfect cusp to fossa arrangement will be a "tripod" contact, consisting of three discrete contacts around the cusp tip for perfect stability. That is a laudable aim, but is difficult to achieve and is often lost as restorations wear.

It is the practitioner's responsibility to prescribe the materials for the occlusal surfaces, recognising that certain combinations of materials can result in excessive wear; for example, ceramic against tooth or metal, particularly if the ceramic has not been polished or reglazed after occlusal adjustments. If materials are poorly selected, the problem of differential wear can occur, causing some occlusal contacts to wear much faster than others, potentially resulting in occlusal instability. Adopting a policy of "like against like" – metal against metal or ceramic against ceramic – is usually sensible. Metal alloys are less damaging to enamel than porcelain.

Achieving occlusal stability is not easy, but it is important. A case in which failure to establish stability resulted in challenging problems is illustrated in Fig 4-6.

Guidance Teeth and Protection from Damage

In addition to providing for stability, the occlusal scheme also defines the way the teeth are shaped to facilitate function and, specifically, guidance. Approaches to guidance under preset occlusal schemes are shown in Table 4-1, but some flexibility is required. The following six points are simple indicators of good practice and common sense with respect to guidance when restorations are being placed during a reorganisation:

- As discussed in Chapter 2, canines are the optimum guidance teeth for lateral excursions, provided they are not compromised periodontally, structurally weakened or restored with non-retentive restorations or post crowns. Under such circumstances, we would suggest transferring guidance to the premolars, or, where possible, creating group function between all of the teeth in the buccal segment.
- Where the canines alone are not going to be used for guidance in lateral excursions, sharing guidance is advisable, but this is sometimes difficult to achieve. This is best delivered by having the technician construct the crowns on a semi-adjustable articulator, so that they can be shaped and adjusted to achieve the desired outcome. Crowns made to provide group function should require minimal, if any, adjustment, provided the clinical records and laboratory work have been carefully undertaken.
- Non-working-side interferences are not in anyone's interest (see Chapter 3). Again, the use of a semi-adjustable articulator for laboratory-made restorations should minimise the risk of incorporating any such interferences in the occlusal scheme.
- Protrusive guidance is usually best shared between the two central incisors with equal contacts in the edge-to-edge position. Crowned lateral incisors are structurally compromised, so if possible make their guidance contacts light. The use of a semi-adjustable articulator during restoration manufacture will help enormously. Where direct composite restorations are used to provide new guidance surfaces, clinical time can be saved if you use a silicone matrix made from a diagnostic wax-up (see Section 8-8) to shape the palatal surfaces.
- Where there are bridge pontics, in particular cantilevers, it is best to avoid any guidance on these. Excursive loading of cantilever pontics can rotate the abutment tooth, dislodge the bridge or even fracture the preparation. Nevertheless, with some fixed–fixed bridges – for example a bridge replacing the four upper incisors using canines as abutments – it is difficult to avoid placing guidance on the pontics. In such cases, great care needs to be taken to ensure guidance is spread evenly and in harmony with mandibular movements.
- To ensure the patient is comfortable with their reorganised occlusion, the concepts of "mutually protected occlusion" and "freedom in centric" are helpful (see Table 4-1). These are less important matters

and not always critical to success, but both achieve a similar goal of allowing the condyles a small amount of anteroposterior movement when the patient bites into their new ICP. Clinically, some patients appear very sensitive to a lack of any anteroposterior movement into their ICP – sometimes described as "locking". To avoid such difficulties, it is always worth ensuring that the new ICP does not incorporate excessively steep cuspal inclines or anterior guidance slopes.

Sometimes it is simply not possible to meet all of the requirements of an ideal occlusion, and you may have to make limited compromises. For example, if many of the teeth are periodontally involved or have little natural tooth tissue remaining, the options for guidance may be limited; while a perfect mutually protected occlusion may be some way from reality in cases in which many teeth are missing. Some compromise is reasonable, but too much can bring into question the long-term viability of the completed case. It is inappropriate to prescribe an expensive rehabilitation that is destined to fail within a year or two of placement.

The Practicalities of Reorganising

Diagnosis and Planning

As every case is unique, planning is something that needs to be individually customised. Information needs are, however, generally the same for all cases. In addition to the blindingly obvious – a detailed charting, pulp tests, appropriate radiographs and photographs – there are some very specific information needs:

- The information from an occlusal examination underpins everything else. It is essential to know what is happening before starting. (Read Section 8-1 and watch DVD video K for details.)
- *Excellent* study casts, *carefully* mounted in CR in a semi-adjustable articulator are generally an essential prerequisite (look at Sections 8-2, 8-4 and 8-5 for details). Use a second set of casts to prepare a diagnostic wax-up, allowing you to work with your laboratory to design and model an appropriate occlusal scheme. This is extraordinarily useful for determining feasibility. It also gives the patient a three-dimensional model of what you intend. Although study casts add to the total costs, cases involving reorganisation, which have many possible pitfalls, are expensive and so proper planning is essential. (The technicalities of diagnostic wax-ups are considered in Section 8-8.)

When the information is in place, the starting conditions are known and the end point clearly visualised (preferably modelled as a diagnostic wax-up), it is then a matter of thinking one's way through the process of how to get from one to the other. As every case is different, the treatment plan must be customised to best suit the patient. Some general guidelines do, however, apply in all cases.

Recognising the Potentially Difficult Case
It is important to recognise at the outset whether the proposed reorganisation is going to be difficult or relatively straightforward. Indicators to help recognise a potentially difficult case include:
- wear associated with heavy parafunctional grinding (Fig 4-5)
- active TMDs (see Chapter 7), in particular those which fail to respond to splint treatment
- a pattern of tooth loss which compromises occlusal stability; for example, a "battlement occlusion", in which there are teeth in both arches but they occlude only against edentulous areas.

Paradoxically, obtaining occlusal stability is usually relatively straightforward in patients with many missing teeth because typically only a few natural teeth require adjustment.

Reorganising with Adhesively Retained Restorations
Increasingly, a variety of adhesive restorations – such as metal, porcelain and composite onlays – are used for occlusal reorganisation. These restorations are less destructive of natural tooth tissue than full-coverage crowns. Directly placed composite restorations can be especially versatile (Fig 4-4), although it is more difficult to achieve occlusal control with direct rather than indirect restorations. With experience, however, excellent results can be achieved. The risk of chipping or bulk fracture of indirect restorations can be minimised by providing an adequate thickness of material – at least 1 mm – and through careful adjustment of the occlusion. A wax-up may be helpful to prescribe the shape of the guidance surfaces. The wax-up can either form a guide for freehand contouring or be used to make putty matrices to shape the lingual and incisal aspects of teeth being built up. Although composites form excellent transitional restorations, it may be necessary to consider replacing such restorations with restorations of metal or porcelain if it is likely that the restored teeth will be subjected to heavy occlusal forces. The advantages of adhesive techniques are considerable, making such an approach an attractive option. For direct composites, it is important to use a hard-wearing hybrid composite and to plan regular reviews.

Treatment Sequencing

Reorganisation rarely involves preparing all the teeth in one arch, let alone in both arches, simultaneously. This is a high-risk strategy appropriate for only a tiny minority of patients. Breaking the work down into a number of manageable stages allows the vast majority of cases to be successfully managed, albeit that it requires a series of appointments. In such cases, provisional restorations are often required to maintain occlusal stability throughout treatment. The importance of ensuring that provisional restorations are of excellent quality is critical.

Although rules are made to be broken, the following sequence may be helpful for completing extensive reorganisations at the same vertical dimension using crowns and bridges:

1. Provide posterior stability first. This involves removing deflective contacts and interferences and providing stable ICP contacts on natural teeth, cores or provisional restorations by means of occlusal adjustment, including the recontouring of existing restorations.
2. Establish anterior guidance on provisional restorations. This typically involves careful adjustment over a period to ensure harmonious contacts and patient comfort.
3. Copy the anterior guidance into the definitive restorations (see Section 8-9 for techniques).
4. Provide definitive posterior restorations.

The same approach can be used in cases in which the vertical dimension is to be changed. Guidelines in respect of the technicalities involved in changing the vertical dimension using different approaches are given in Section 8-11. For guidelines on articulator selection see Section 8-6.

Conclusions

Reorganising the occlusion is not something to be undertaken lightly, but equally it is not something to have anxieties about. The option to reorganise opens up possibilities for stable, long-lasting treatments. Occlusal reorganisation is a precise art based on three very specific principles: building the occlusion around a reproducible jaw position, achieving an appropriate vertical dimension and providing an appropriate occlusal scheme. The choice of occlusal scheme has been the topic of heated debate over many years, with little underlying evidence. Nevertheless, there are some simple rules that help to design final restorations that will achieve stability, harmony and protection of the occlusion. Finally, never start treatment before completing planning; always seek advice if you think you need it.

Further Reading

Becker CM, Kaiser DA. Evolution of occlusion and occlusal instruments. J Prosthodont 1993:2;33–43.

Redman CD, Hemmings KW, Good JA. The survival and clinical performance of resin-based composite restorations used to treat localised anterior tooth wear. Br Dent J 2003;194:566–572; discussion 559.

Wassell RW, Steele JG, Welsh G. Considerations when planning occlusal rehabilitation: a review of the literature. Int Dent J 1998;48:571–581.

Wassell RW, St George G, Ingledew RP, Steele JG. Crowns and other extra-coronal restorations: provisional restorations. Br Dental J 2002;192:619–622, 625–630.

Chapter 5

Occlusion, the Periodontium and Soft Tissues

Aim

The aims of this chapter are to:
- explore the relationship between occlusion and increased tooth mobility, with or without reduced periodontal support
- discuss possible links between occlusion and periodontal disease
- consider soft tissue damage, such as lip, cheek and tongue biting, related to adverse tooth/tissue relationships.

Outcome

At the end of this chapter, the clinician should:
- be aware of the occlusal causes for tooth mobility and tooth migration
- know when occlusal adjustment is indicated for mobile teeth
- comprehend the relationship between occlusion and periodontal disease
- recognise when occlusal factors may contribute to tooth positional relapse after orthodontics
- appreciate how incorrect restoration design can contribute to lip, cheek and tongue biting.

Occlusal Trauma Related to the Periodontium

Mobile and drifting teeth often distress patients. They cause discomfort, difficulty with chewing and aesthetic problems. Practitioners need to be aware of these problems, understand their causes and be able to provide possible solutions. First, though, it is important to be able to measure tooth mobility and understand its significance. Although devices exist to quantify tooth mobility very precisely, in everyday practice we normally rely on rather crude clinical judgement, such as the current version of the Miller classification (Table 5-1), where the handles of two instruments are used to move the tooth under examination in a buccolingual direction.

The term "fremitus" describes tooth mobility when occlusal contacts are performed. It may either be observed visually or felt through the examiner's fingertips, or both. It may occur when the patient closes into the intercuspal or retruded positions, or during excursions of the mandible.

Occlusal factors may be important in the aetiology of increased mobility, but there are often other reasons. These are considered in the following section. Where the occlusion interacts with these factors, it may worsen or prevent resolution of the mobility. An increased mobility associated primarily to occlusal overload is relatively uncommon, but it can mystify the unwary dentist, particularly when it affects multiple teeth.

Non-occlusally Related Causes for Tooth Hypermobility

The commonest cause of increased tooth mobility is inflammatory periodontal disease. All clinicians are aware that teeth tighten after successful periodontal treatment, but increased mobility can persist after the inflammation has been eliminated. Characteristically, radiographs of affected teeth show reduced alveolar support, but a normal periodontal ligament space. This is simply an amplification of physiological mobility (Fig 5-1) because of long clinical crown height and short attachment. Despite the apparent increased mobility, such teeth do not require occlusal treatment if not subject to occlusal interference.

Table 5-1 **The Miller classification of tooth mobility**

Class	Mobility
0	no detectable movement
I	<1 mm buccolingually
II	1–2 mm buccolingually
III	>2 mm buccolingually and/or vertically

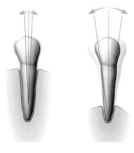

Fig 5-1 Although the tooth on the right is more mobile than the tooth on the left, the periodontal ligament is healthy and not widened. The increased mobility at the level of the occlusal plane is simply related to the longer clinical crown.

Only if the patient has discomfort from excessively hypermobile teeth during function, or if the mobility is increasing, might splinting be beneficial.

Other non-occlusal causes of increased mobility include:
- root resorption
- loss of periradicular bone support, for example due to periradicular inflammation or after apical surgery
- recent trauma causing subluxation
- fractured root
- hormonal, occurring occasionally during pregnancy.

Occlusally Related Causes for Tooth Hypermobility

Habits such as bruxism can subject the teeth to loads which are higher and longer lasting than during normal function. This may, for poorly understood reasons, result in the periodontium adapting to the increased loads, rather than the neuromuscular system limiting load generation, as might be expected. Teeth with normal bone levels and normal attachment can still become hypermobile under such circumstances, with the response regarded as a physiological reaction to the mechanical insult. This is sometimes called "primary occlusal trauma". Characteristically, the periodontal ligament becomes widened (Figs 5-2 and 5-3).

The same physiological response of the periodontium can occur where there has been some change in the occlusal scheme, resulting in adversely changed

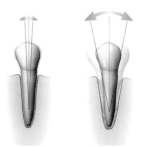

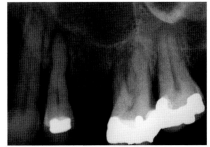

Fig 5-2 The tooth on the right shows the physiological response to a higher than normal occlusal force; its periodontal ligament has become widened (primary occlusal trauma).

Fig 5-3 A premolar with a widened periodontal ligament space. This is periodontal ligament widening, caused in this case by abnormal loading from a denture clasp.

loading, often non-axially directed. The increase in mobility can affect an individual tooth or a group of teeth. This might happen when a new restoration produces a premature occlusal contact or interference (direct occlusal trauma), or as a result of an occlusal interference somewhere else in the mouth causing a damaging deflection (indirect occlusal trauma). These problems are well illustrated in the DVD animations E, F and G. The same underlying mechanisms can sometimes explain migration of teeth and tooth positional relapse following orthodontic treatment (see the section Pathological Tooth Migration, below). 🔘E 🔘F 🔘G

Of course, teeth with a reduced but healthy periodontal support may undergo an increase in existing hypermobility if subjected to direct or indirect occlusal trauma. This is sometimes called "secondary occlusal trauma". This terminology is not useful because the response to both primary and secondary occlusal trauma simply represents a normal physiological adaptation of the periodontium to increased occlusal loading.

A thorough clinical and radiographic examination will enable the cause of hypermobility to be identified. Increasing mobility is an important clinical symptom and sign to look out for. It can indicate an occlusal discrepancy which will benefit from correction.

In addition to conventional periodontal therapy, management of hypermobility caused by occlusal factors should be directed at:
• attempting to reduce bruxing behaviours, or at least to protect the teeth from damage using an occlusal splint (see Section 8-10)
• investigating the feasibility of occlusal adjustment, if there are associated interferences or steep excursive contacts; this is especially important if the interferences are additionally preventing comfortable function or are thought to be of importance to the aetiology of a concurrent temporomandibular disorder (TMD) (see Chapter 7 regarding occlusal factors and TMD and Section 8-7) – the message here is that if there is problematic increased mobility, it is worth looking for an occlusal cause
• splinting teeth together to reduce discomfort associated with function on hypermobile teeth; this may take the form of a fixed or removable device.

The Relationship between Occlusion and Periodontal Disease

Can occlusal factors influence the initiation or progression of plaque-induced periodontal disease? This question has long been debated and many human and animal studies have been undertaken in attempt to answer it.

Most animal studies have investigated the effect of so-called "jiggling" forces produced by introducing occlusal interferences. Occlusal trauma to the healthy periodontium with either normal or reduced bone levels (i.e. after treatment of periodontitis) has been shown to cause an initial progressive increase in mobility which then stabilised. Although there was a widened periodontal ligament, there was no pocket formation or loss of connective tissue attachment. In other words, a normal physiological adaptation occurred. Following occlusal correction, the increased mobility and widening of the periodontal ligament resolved within a matter of 2 weeks.

Occlusal trauma in the presence of plaque-induced periodontitis caused accelerated pocket formation in beagle dogs. However, the same occlusal trauma in squirrel monkeys caused bone loss but no loss of attachment, possibly suggesting a species-related response. In human studies, the evidence is not conclusive and investigations are fraught with difficulties, not least that it would be unethical to carry out a randomised controlled prospective study in volunteers.

What can be said is that trauma from occlusion cannot by itself induce periodontal breakdown. Most clinicians take the pragmatic view that occlusal trauma or occlusal interference is a risk factor (or co-factor) for accelerated attachment loss in pre-existing plaque-induced periodontal disease. Occlusally mediated hypermobility should be managed as outlined in the previous section, but only after primary treatment for periodontal disease.

Pathological Tooth Migration

Pathological tooth migration (PTM) is defined as a change in tooth position that occurs when there is disruption of the forces that maintain teeth in a normal relationship. Patients commonly present being troubled by progressively enlarging anterior interdental spaces (Fig 5-4). Although PTM is most common in patients with attachment loss caused by periodontal disease, occlusal factors alone can be responsible for this condition. In combination with periodontal disease, occlusal factors substantially increase the risk of PTM. Several interacting occlusal factors may be responsible:

• **Loss of stable posterior occlusal stability:** This may be encountered in the severely shortened dental arch. A reduced dental arch may be a factor predisposing to PTM, as occlusal forces are distributed more anteriorly. Both periodontal disease and bruxism may exacerbate the situation.

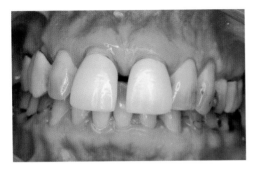

Fig 5-4 Pathological tooth migration. In this case the cause is a combination of destruction to periodontal support by periodontal disease and replacement crowns with pronounced palatal contours forming occlusal interference in protrusion.

- **Loss of arch integrity:** If interproximal contacts are lost, the distribution of occlusal forces is likely to change, predisposing to PTM.
- **Class II malocclusion:** Incisor proclination with non-axial distribution of occlusal forces may help to explain why PTM is more common in patients with proclined teeth (Fig 5-5). Of course, soft-tissue factors such as lip entrapment also need to be taken into account.
- **Posterior occlusal interferences:** These can cause the mandible to be deflected anteriorly, subjecting the incisors to forces which may cause PTM (see DVD animation G). Overeruption of anterior teeth diagonally opposite a posterior non-working-side occlusal interference has also been observed. 🄖
- **Anterior component of force:** Occlusal function produces a component of force that is projected anteriorly by interproximal contacts. This may account for PTM if the force is not resisted by such factors as a healthy periodontium and competent lip morphology. People who brux may be susceptible to this cause of PTM, even if they have a healthy periodontium.

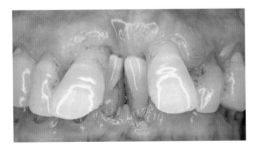

Fig 5-5 A Class II incisor relation combined with occlusal collapse. Periodontal disease has resulted in unsightly opening of a large median diastema.

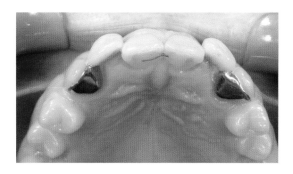

Fig 5-6 Mild relapse in the relationship of the canines towards the positions they occupied before orthodontic realignment has caused the lateral incisor cantilevered pontics to swing outwards to an unacceptable degree.

- **Protrusive pattern mastication:** Studies of mandibular movement have identified that some people have a protrusive pattern of mastication. This could account for PTM and attrition of anterior teeth.
- **Bruxism and parafunction:** It is easy to understand how excessive occlusal forces or forces acting for longer than normal and in abnormal directions may cause PTM.
- **Post-orthodontic movement:** The positions occupied by teeth after they have been moved orthodontically are inherently unstable. Teeth which have been derotated are especially prone to so-called "orthodontic relapse" (Fig 5-6).

The occlusal and periodontal factors which predispose to tooth mobility and pathological tooth migration may contribute to any tendency to relapse after orthodontic treatment. For example, steepening the guidance on an anterior tooth which has previously been retracted by, for example, attaching an adhesive bridge retainer may be enough to produce the sort of occlusal interference that will encourage positional relapse. This creates a dilemma: whether to use bridgework of fixed–fixed design to replace missing teeth where the abutments have been moved orthodontically, or to opt for a cantilever design, which may impart no inherent tooth positional stability but which may have less chance of cement failure. The limited amount of research in this area suggests that fixed–fixed is the design of choice in these specific circumstances, provided an adequate area for adhesive bonding is available. Advice about tendency to relapse and post-treatment retention should be sought from the orthodontist.

Direct Occlusal Damage to Soft Tissues

It is not uncommon for cheeks, lips or tongue to become traumatised when the teeth come into contact. This may be caused by sharp tooth or restoration margins catching the tissues as they slide past. If there is little or no buccal overjet, the tendency for this to happen is more likely, notably with posterior teeth. Occasionally, patients bite their cheeks or lips because of mandibular incoordination as they close to avoid a posterior deflective contact. Alternatively, patients may chew the soft tissues as part of a parafunctional habit. Whatever the reason, once traumatised the tissues swell, making it likely that they will be subject to further trauma.

A deep overbite can also be associated with periodontal lesions. The classic picture is where the mandibular incisors contact the palatal gingival margins of the maxillary teeth and there is inflammation, recession or both (Fig 5-7). It is easy to appreciate how this incisor relationship may predispose to food impaction and gingival inflammation, possibly creating the environment for localised periodontal destruction. It is also possible that the traumatised appearance of the mucosa is the result of localised gingival inflammation (perhaps as a consequence of hygiene difficulties palatal to retroclined teeth), with the swollen tissue becoming indented by the opposing teeth. A vicious cycle can become established whereby discomfort prevents effective oral hygiene, and with inflammation occlusal trauma develops. Accordingly, efforts to resolve any inflammation must be instituted as the first line of treatment in such situations.

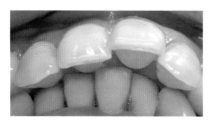

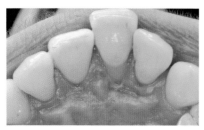

Fig 5-7 The mandibular incisors impinge onto the palatal mucosa just behind the maxillary incisors. There are areas of palatal indentation (Ackerly Type I incisor relationship) and areas of palatal recession (Akerly Type II).

Non-surgical periodontal management is often sufficient, otherwise treatment for this problem can be difficult. Sometimes, periodic use of a removable appliance that protects the soft tissues from direct contact with the opposing teeth will suffice. Occasionally, it is possible to create new stable interincisal contacts and harmonious anterior guidance by using fixed restorations to recontour the maxillary incisors. This is often very difficult or unpredictable. Removable appliances can also be used to create the same stabilising occlusal features.

For both approaches, interocclusal space is often lacking, so manoeuvres to create this have to be devised (see Section 8-11). Orthodontic realignment and/or orthognathic surgery may be considered to correct what is often an underlying malocclusion, including the deep "traumatic" overbite. These cases are very difficult and some degree of compromise is often necessary.

We find the Ackerly classification useful to categorise incisor relationships in relation to the possible associations with both hard- and soft-tissue damage (Table 5-2).

Table 5-2 **The Ackerly classification**

Class	Description
I	Mandibular incisors contact the palatal mucosa away from the vicinity of the maxillary palatal gingival margins. May manifest as discomfort or indentation
II	Often a Class II div. i incisor relationship, where the mandibular incisors contact the palatal gingival margins of the maxillary teeth. May manifest as inflammation (and recession) at the maxillary palatal gingival margins
III	Class II div. ii incisor relationship, where the mandibular incisors contact the palatal gingival margins of the maxillary teeth and the maxillary incisors contact the labial gingival margins of the mandibular teeth. May manifest as inflammation (and recession) at the maxillary palatal and mandibular labial gingival margins
IV	Class I or II div. i incisor relationship, associated with wear facets on the palatal surface of maxillary teeth and/or labial surfaces of mandibular teeth

Conclusions

The important message from this chapter is not to assume that all tooth mobility is the result of loss of periodontal attachment linked to periodontal disease. Careful clinical and radiographic examination facilitates the diagnosis of occlusally mediated tooth mobility and leads the way to appropriate management.

Further Reading

Akerly WB. Prosthodontic treatment of traumatic overlap of the anterior teeth. J Prosthet Dent 1977;38:26–34.

Brunsvold M. Pathologic tooth migration. J Periodontol 2005;76:859–866.

Davies SJ, Gray RJM, Linden GJ, James JA. Occlusal considerations in periodontics. Br Dent J. 2001;191:597–604.

Gher ME. Changing concepts – the effects of occlusion on periodontitis. Dent Clin N Am 1998;42:285–297.

Nasry HA, Barclay SC. Periodontal lesions associated with deep traumatic overbite. Br Dent J 2006;200:557–561.

Chapter 6
Occlusion and Fixed Osseointegrated Implant Restorations

Aim

The aims of this chapter are to consider relevant factors during the planning, placement and maintenance of fixed restorations retained by implants and to emphasise the differences between osseointegrated implants and natural teeth in relation to occlusion.

Outcome

At the end of this chapter, the clinician should:
- be aware of causes of mechanical failure of implants or superstructure components
- appreciate occlusally related factors in planning an implant case, namely:
  - influence of parafunction
  - space for restoration
  - problems of non-axial loading
  - vulnerability of cantilevered pontics
  - indications for linking implant restorations together
  - problems of linking implants and teeth together
- know which occlusal schemes are appropriate in planning for implants
- be aware of the occlusal factors to take into account in both immediate and early implant loading.

This chapter will help in treatment planning and in troubleshooting occlusal causes of implant complications. Some aspects of the relationship between implants and occlusion are not yet "evidenced based", so clinical decisions often depend on sound common sense and applied clinical experience.

Implants Compared with Natural Teeth

The fundamental difference between teeth and implants is that teeth have a periodontal ligament whereas implants are rigidly attached to bone. This may sound obvious, but this simple fact underpins all of the specific considerations for implant occlusion. The periodontal ligament is an evolutionary triumph.

It is highly sensate, able to detect an object finer than a human hair, it acts as a shock absorber and it allows for adaptive occlusal changes. The increase in mobility and drifting in response to heavy occlusal loads described in the previous chapter are simply a reflection of how these adaptive changes have a protective function in the face of occlusal overload. Osseointegrated dental implants do not have these protective mechanisms. The osseointegration between bone and implant may be a feat of human ingenuity, but it is a poor match for the versatility of the periodontal ligament. Implant-retained restorations are therefore potentially at greater risk from occlusal damage than are natural teeth (Table 6-1).

An example of how the biological difference between the periodontal ligament and the osseointegration interface may affect occlusal management can be found at the very simplest level. When asking a dentate patient to help locate restoration high spots on a natural tooth they can often do this quite easily, and give an indication of how much more adjustment is still required. For restorations on implants, there will still be some proprioception mediated by receptors in the periosteum, muscles of mastication, oral mucosa and temporomandibular joints, but in the absence of the periodontal ligament even a straightforward adjustment can be more demanding, relying entirely on the clinician's ability to detect very small differences in contact.

Combining natural teeth, with their adaptive capacity and protective mechanisms, together with rigid implants in the same arch is associated with particular problems. Taking out natural teeth of dubious prognosis and replacing them with an implant-retained prosthesis is sometimes an attractive option, but it will result in loss of proprioception and an increased risk of occlusal damage. Consequently, leaving natural teeth in the arch to provide

Table 6-1 **Risks to osseointegrated implants from occlusal overload**

• Failure of integration at the bone–implant interface, leading to eventual implant loosening and loss
• Implant fracture

• Mechanical failure of any of implant superstructure stack:
  – abutment screw
  – prosthetic screw
  – crown/bridge superstructure

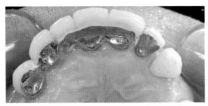 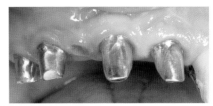

Fig 6-1 The superstructure borne by implants at UR4, UR3, UR1, UL1 has been linked together with the aim of distributing excursive occlusal loads to all the implants. UL2 carries a gold palatal veneer, enabling it to be "recruited" into occlusal contact, thus providing a degree of protection for the implant superstructure.

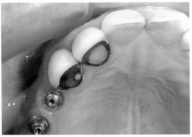 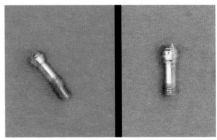

Fig 6-2 This patient presented with two abutment screw fractures, which were preceded by increased mobility of the crowned teeth at UR2 and UR3, possibly resulting from parafunctional habits. As a result, it is conceivable that the implant crowns, which were previously protected from excursive contacts, had become exposed to increased non-axial loading.

some protective proprioception has its attractions (Fig 6-1). On the other hand, if there is a parafunctional habit or reduced periodontal support for the natural teeth they may drift, leaving the implant restorations to take all of the load anyway. Such a case is shown in Fig 6-2. Where there is such damaging parafunction, protection with an occlusal splint is advisable. Deciding how to manage such situations is not always easy. In fact, joining teeth and implants together in a single restoration is potentially even more problematic. These issues will be considered in detail later in this chapter.

Planning the Foundations of Implant Occlusion

The key to successful planning of implant numbers and positions is to think "tooth-down". To put it another way, it is crucial to establish the aesthetic and occlusal form of the proposed implant superstructure before carrying out surgery, whether to place an implant or even to augment a proposed implant site. Only when the planning has been successfully completed can an informed decision be made about whether sufficient hard and soft tissue are available in the most favourable location in which to place an implant. Determining the final occlusal scheme (implants need an occlusal scheme too; see Chapter 4) is a critical part of the planning process and should be considered right at the outset along with aesthetics, phonetics, the load-bearing capacity of the implant–bone interface and a range of other considerations.

Early in the assessment, it is necessary to establish whether there is sufficient interocclusal space to accommodate the implant superstructure, including the crown. In the posterior regions this is relatively easy to assess (Fig 6-3), but anteriorly it can be more difficult (Fig 6-4).

The important thing is to envisage the ideal volume to be filled by the final implant-borne restoration, taking into account the overjet and overbite. This

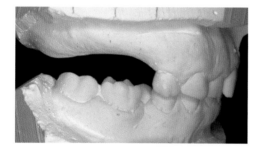

Fig 6-3 The interocclusal space available for a maxillary implant superstructure is clearly visible between these study casts held in ICP.

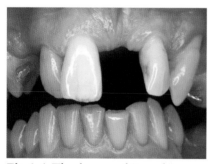
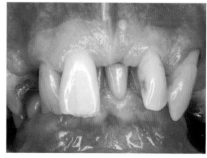

Fig 6-4 The deep overbite and presence of an overjet make assessment of space for an implant superstructure difficult.

is sometimes, rather aptly, called the "prosthetic envelope" and it is easiest to evaluate using a diagnostic wax-up (Fig 6-5).

The precise minimum interocclusal distances required will depend on the implant system used and whether the restoration is screw or cement retained. Screw-retained restorations are more retrievable and may require less occlusal clearance than cemented ones because there is no need for preparation height. A wax-up also allows for detailed planning of a conformative or reorganised approach to managing the occlusion.

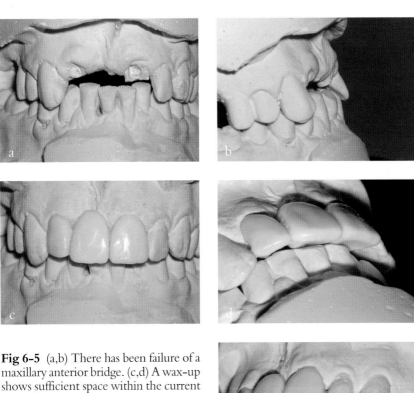

Fig 6-5 (a,b) There has been failure of a maxillary anterior bridge. (c,d) A wax-up shows sufficient space within the current ICP for a bridge superstructure borne by implants at UR2 and UL1. (e) Examination of excursive movements with casts on a semi-adjustable articulator showing disclusion of the proposed implant bridge with left lateral excursion carried by the existing natural teeth.

Avoiding Non-axial Loading

Ideally, implants should direct occlusal loads axially into the supporting bone, but some level of compromise is often necessary; for example:

- an implant which has to be placed with an exaggerated angulated trajectory relative to the general long axis of the tooth or teeth being replaced (Fig 6-6)
- having an implant exposed to cantilevered occlusal loads given an unfavourable position or small diameter, or because the implant carries a cantilever pontic (Fig 6-7)
- there may have to be a crown to implant length ratio of more than 1:1 (Fig 6-8).

In day-to-day clinical practice, dentists often accept such compromises (either by design or by accident) with remarkably few apparent complications. Nevertheless, there is evidence of a greater risk of mechanical failure of implant–superstructure assemblies subjected to the damaging tensile and shear stresses of non-axial loads. Such evidence comes from clinical experience and from bench-top and animal experiments. It is, therefore, better to avoid non-axial loading scenarios if you can.

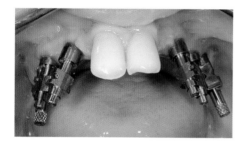

Fig 6-6 Despite bone augmentation it was necessary in this case to accept buccal trajectory of several implants, which are shown carrying impression copings. This patient has multiple congenitally absent teeth. The implants were ultimately linked by cemented bridges.

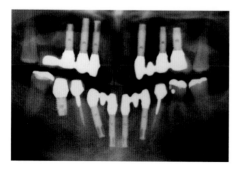

Fig 6-7 Linked implants in the upper right quadrant support a cantilevered pontic where further implant placement was not possible. This patient had already undergone sinus floor bone augmentation to allow implants to be placed that have sufficient length to support a posterior cantilever.

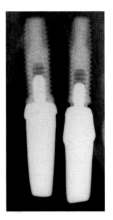

Fig 6-8 Unfavourable crown to implant ratio. The lever arm effect of the crowns in function risks mechanical failure of components or failure of osseointegration. One of the abutments in this radiograph is clearly not fitting the implant and needs to be rectified before the abutment screw is fully tightened.

Cantilevered Restorations

Ideally, implants should be placed to give a broad distribution of loading directly beneath the fixed restorations, but the reality is that there is often inadequate bone in key areas. As a consequence, cantilevered pontics are used. Indeed, cantilevers are a feature of implant-supported restoration design in the edentulous mandible. The implant-bearing area lies between the two mental foramina and the framework is usually cantilevered distally above the inferior dental nerve. Similarly, in the edentulous maxilla, the maxillary sinuses may prevent implant placement, unless they are augmented surgically. In fact, in the maxilla, which is also subject to facial resorption after tooth loss, the framework may have to have cantilevered extensions both posteriorly and anteriorly. Because the quality of the bone is relatively poor in the maxilla, very careful planning of implant numbers and locations is required, particularly if cantilever extensions are planned. Further guidelines on judging the dimensions of cantilever extensions and implant positions and numbers can be found in the list of further reading (Jivraj et al., 2006).

Where cantilevers are prescribed, the implants themselves need to be sufficiently long and well integrated into sound bone to carry non-axial loading, even when linked together (Fig 6-7). In an edentulous jaw, the arch form of the fixed prosthesis helps distribute stresses between the implants. In a part-dentate jaw, such cross-arch stabilisation is often not possible, resulting in the need for greater caution with shorter sectional restorations carrying cantilevers. In the posterior maxilla, where there is doubt over the bone's load-bearing capacity it is probably better to avoid distal cantilevering completely where possible.

Linking Implants

Notwithstanding the need to link implants for cantilevered pontics, there are other situations where implants may need to be linked to share occlusal loads – both static and dynamic. Linking is generally safe, as implants are effectively ankylosed and do not move; in contrast, bridgework supported by multiple teeth is at risk of decementation due to root movements within the periodontal ligament. In linking implants there may be implications for aesthetics, hygiene and technical achievability. The following factors favour linking implants:

- Posterior maxillary implants where loads are high and bone is of relatively low density.
- Implants in grafted bone, in particular in posterior regions of the jaws.
- Where steep excursive contacts on implants are unavoidable.
- Short, small-diameter implants, notably those involved with excursive contacts.
- Where implants are used to support cantilevered pontics.
- Patients who show evidence or a history of attritive tooth wear or bruxing. In such cases it is likely that occlusal contacts are more frequent or loads are higher than normal. As mentioned earlier in this chapter, an occlusal splint is recommended for nocturnal wear.

If implants are to be linked in the posterior regions, there is merit in taking the opportunity to distribute them off-axis, thus maximising any cantilever load-bearing capacity (Fig 6-9). Linking implants also has the practical advantage of not having to adjust interproximal contacts at the time of fit. Screw-retained linked prostheses require perfect passive fit, otherwise stresses will be introduced into the implant superstructure and bone–implant interface at the time of screw tightening. These stresses may not only compromise the occlusal outcome, but also result in mechanical failure (e.g. porcelain fracture).

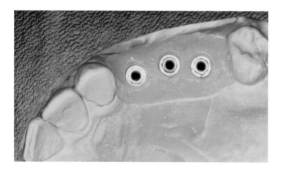

Fig 6-9 These three implants do not lie in a straight line, which means they are better able to withstand non-axial loads.

Linking Implants to Teeth

On theoretical grounds, this arrangement is unfavourable because of the different support mechanisms for implants and teeth. Breakage of implant components, damage to abutment teeth or intrusion of abutment teeth are all possible. Movable connections have been employed in an attempt to accommodate the difference in support. However, after a 5-year period, intrusion may be detected in about 5% of abutment teeth – typically teeth with non-rigid attachment to implants, illustrating graphically the adaptive capacity of the periodontal ligament.

Despite the potential problems of differential support and tooth intrusion, it is possible to link teeth to implants with satisfactory results using either rigid or non-rigid connection. The advice here would be to proceed with caution and to use this approach in fallback situations. In the unusual event of implant failure, or the inability to place implants in their planned positions, linking to teeth can be an acceptable alternative. The evidence suggests that rigid connection is a better alternative than non-rigid connection, at least with respect to tooth intrusion.

Having considered aspects of implant placement and occlusal loading, it is important to focus on the pattern of occlusal contact developed on the restorations – the occlusal scheme.

Idealised Occlusal Schemes

With fixed implant-retained restorations there are differences in managing the occlusion depending on whether they are being used to restore a partly dentate or an edentulous jaw. In both cases it is helpful to think of the static and dynamic occlusal scenarios, either conforming with the existing occlusion or reorganising it, in exactly the same way as we do with natural teeth (see Chapter 4). However, the basic rules are slightly different.

Partly Dentate Jaw

One of the first decisions to be made after evaluating the restorative space, supporting tissues and prosthesis design is whether to work conformatively or to reorganise the occlusion. Working conformatively essentially means that you accept the existing dental occlusion, perhaps with some minor modification; for example, reduction of overerupted teeth, elimination of interferences (especially on teeth that are to be restored) or building guidance surfaces strategically to reduce loading on implants during lateral excursions. You may need to consider reorganising the occlusion in cases in which the existing ICP is unstable, where deflective contacts cause an anterior thrust, or where restorative space can be achieved either by increasing the vertical dimension or, more rarely, by eliminating the horizontal component of slide between the retruded contact position and ICP. This is no different from a natural dentition. With the exception of the points made below, the patterns of occlusal contact within reorganised occlusions are similar whether the reconstruction involves teeth or implants. These are discussed in Chapter 4.

Static occlusion
In partially dentate patients, teeth will move to a small degree in their sockets under occlusal loading. Great care must be taken with implant restorations, which are rigid, to avoid occlusal overload. The recommendation is that implant crowns should have a 30 μm clearance in heavy clenching. To put this in perspective, shim-stock foil is about 10 μm thick; the patient should be able to grip three layers of shim, but two should pull through. This sounds very precise but it gives an indication of the attention to detail required where no periodontal ligament is present.

Dynamic occlusion
Keeping excursive contacts on healthy natural teeth, with their inherent proprioceptive capacity, makes sound prosthodontic sense. This feature is often seen to be present (Fig 6-5). On the other hand, scrutiny of a diagnostic wax-up produced on casts articulated using a facebow on a semi-adjustable articulator might show that, despite there being adequate space for an implant restoration in the static position, excursion immediately brings the opposing teeth into steep guidance on the proposed implant restoration, and with it the risk of potentially damaging non-axial loading. If inherent occlusal protection is absent, it may be possible to "recruit" occlusal protection by altering excursive contacts on existing natural teeth to achieve disclusion of the proposed implant crowns (Fig 6-1).

Once again, the difference in support between implants and teeth dictates, where feasible, that there should be excursive clearance on implants of about 30 μm. This can be quite difficult and time consuming to achieve by chair-side refinements. However, given the extent and expense of the treatment, it is a goal worth pursuing.

Where excursive contact on a single implant crown or multiple implant crowns is unavoidable, it makes sense that the guidance should be shallow to minimise non-axial loading, in particular in the posterior regions where forces are relatively high.

Edentulous Jaw

Static occlusion

As there are no teeth to provide ICP, you need to reorganise using the temporomandibular joints as the starting point (centric relation), around which the new contacts are built at the desired vertical dimension. This approach is discussed in Chapter 4. It is not really any different to the procedure for constructing a complete denture. Cantilever extensions often feature as part of fixed-restoration design. To avoid occlusal overload, such extensions require a clearance of 30 μm; this particularly applies to distal cantilevers, which are especially vulnerable to excessive loading.

Dynamic occlusion

The excursive contacts should provide shallow guidance with posterior disclusion. Canine guidance is the easiest way of providing lateral excursion, but, where the canine replacements are not in suitable positions or you need to distribute parafunctional loads, group function may be preferable.

Trial by Temporary

Provisional restorations are very useful in determining the final occlusal design features. Fracture or cement failures with provisional restorations, or possibly the onset of temporomandibular dysfunction, are warning signs that either the static or dynamic occlusion is not functioning adequately. As with the provision of any fixed prosthesis, changes to the dynamic occlusion must be assessed and corrected in the provisional phase before being replicated in the final restorations. Where the width of the occlusal table is narrowed in an effort to reduce masticatory loading (Fig 6-10), care must be taken to ensure sufficient occlusal stability against opposing teeth or restorations.

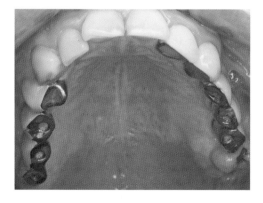

Fig 6-10 The occlusal width of the screw-retained linked implant superstructures in this patient have been reduced in an attempt to limit occlusal loading during function. Care must be taken to avoid loss of occlusal stability in such circumstances.

Immediate and Early Loading

It is easy to understand the attraction to both patient and clinician of reaching the end of treatment as quickly as possible, particularly if this avoids the need for additional surgery. Placing restorations on implants either at the time of placement or in the early weeks during healing has become fairly common practice, with a growing evidence base. It is still not a gold standard, however, and carries risks. Managing the occlusion appropriately in the early stages of treatment is critical to success. All protocols for immediate or early loading aim to avoid or control potentially damaging loads on the implants by, for example, linking implants together or avoiding any kind of occlusal contact (so called "aesthetic loading").

Teamwork

Surgeons often place implants and then pass the case on to another dentist for provision of the implant superstructure. This arrangement can work well, but success relies on a team approach, in particular to planning, which should also include the involvement of the technician. The importance of agreeing clear responsibilities for each member of the team cannot be over-emphasised.

Despite best efforts and the use of preformed surgical stents, it is inevitable that, on occasion, the unexpected will be encountered at the time of implant placement. The implant surgeon must have an excellent working knowledge of the implant system being used, implant occlusion, bone augmentation techniques, and aesthetics. It is often necessary to make decisions at the time of surgery which will have a critical bearing on the outcome of the case. Failure to achieve effective team working can result in costly disappointment and frustration for all concerned.

Maintenance

Changes in occlusion can occur in clinical service for a number of reasons, including wear of teeth and restorations, tooth migration precipitated by periodontal disease, and tooth loss. As outlined at the start of this chapter, there is a risk, notably with parafunction, that the carefully designed and adjusted implant occlusion may alter to one that is potentially damaging to the integrity of the implants (Fig 6-2). Monitoring changes in occlusion and subsequent adjustment, as indicated clinically, are important parts of the ongoing care. Patients should be counselled at the outset of treatment that such monitoring is necessary, possibly together with the provision of a stabilisation splint to protect the dentition from parafunctional forces.

Conclusions

We have emphasised the important differences between periodontally supported teeth and ankylosed implants. These reflect both on the way the occlusion is developed on implant-supported restorations and decisions regarding the placement of implants and superstructure design so that occlusal loads can be transmitted successfully.

Reference

Jivraj S, Chee W, Corrado P. Treatment planning of the edentulous maxilla. Br Dent J 2006;201:261–279.

Further Reading

Pjetursson BE, Tan K, Lang NP, Bragger U, Egger M, Zwahlen M. A systematic review of the survival and complication rates of fixed partial dentures (FPDs) after an observation period of at least 5 years. Clin Oral Implants Res 2004;15:667–676.

Taylor TD, Wiens J, Carr A. Evidence-based considerations for removable prosthodontic and dental implant occlusion: a literature review. J Prosthet Dent 2005;94: 555–560.

Chapter 7
Occlusion and Temporomandibular Disorders

Aim

The aim of this chapter is to consider how occlusion may contribute to temporomandibular disorders (TMDs) while emphasising the importance of TMD diagnosis.

Outcome

At the end of this chapter, the clinician should:
- know the signs and symptoms of TMDs while also understanding the multifactorial origin of these conditions
- appreciate that these signs and conditions are relatively common in the general population
- comprehend the nature of the uncertain relationship between occlusion and TMDs
- be able to screen for TMDs in patients requiring restorative treatment
- be aware of how to diagnose TMDs in patients with jaw problems and facial pain
- understand how and why occlusal splints and occlusal adjustment can be used to manage TMDs.

Introduction

The term TMDs describes a group of conditions with similar signs and symptoms that affect the temporomandibular joints (TMJs), the muscles of mastication, or both. In approximate order of importance, the signs and symptoms of TMDs are:
- pain and tenderness in and around the TMJs and muscles of mastication
- limitation and incoordination of jaw movement
- joint sounds – clicking and crepitus (grating of the joint)
- headaches (increased frequency and severity)
- tinnitus (occasional association).

Function usually makes symptoms worse, so patients may have difficulty eating or simply talking. A common misconception is that problems with the occlusion are a principal cause of TMDs. Although this may be true for a small proportion of patients, it is not for the vast majority. Nevertheless, there is the potential for an occlusal component to TMDs. This will be discussed later in this chapter. Of real practical importance, TMDs must not be aggravated, let alone overlooked, when providing dental treatment. Before considering these aspects of TMDs, it is worth considering some background.

TMD Background

Signs and symptoms of TMDs occur commonly in the general population, but these are generally of little significance. For instance, around 20% of subjects experience TMJ clicking, but this causes problems for only a few.

Despite extensive research, the aetiology of any given patient's TMD often remains unclear. We know from epidemiological studies that it often starts in the mid to late teens, but it can present at almost any age. In the general population, there are slightly more females than males with signs and symptoms of TMD. By contrast, in the population attending hospital TMD clinics, the female to male ratio often exceeds 4:1 and there is some evidence that there may be hormonal influences. There are also other influences, including psychosocial factors associated with stress and chronic pain behaviour, but the relationship between pain and psychosocial factors is not straightforward. There is certainly a link between stress-induced parafunctional activity (bruxism) and muscle-related hypertonicity and TMDs. Conversely, there are also many people without TMD symptoms who habitually grind their teeth.

In some patients, symptoms of TMD follow trauma. In others it starts following a change to the occlusion. Interestingly, recent research suggests there are genetic predispositions to TMDs related to the biochemistry of pain experience. This may eventually help to explain why some people are susceptible to TMDs while others are not. There is no single cause of TMDs; they are multifactorial, with factors that clinically appear to:
• predispose the patient to TMDs – genetic, hormonal, anatomical
• precipitate TMDs – trauma, occlusal changes, parafunction
• prolong TMDs – parafunction and psychological stress.

Individual factors, such as parafunction, may even fall into more than one of these categories. Although signs and symptoms of TMD occur commonly in otherwise healthy subjects, there appears to be a greater prevalence in certain systemic conditions, such as fibromyalgia, systemic joint laxity and rheumatoid arthritis. Fibromyalgia is a condition characterised by generalised muscle pain, including masticatory muscle pain. Patients with systemic joint laxity have a collagen defect, predisposing them to strained ligaments. This may, in turn, result in a disc displacement within the TMJ. With rheumatoid arthritis patients, around half experience arthritic TMJ pain. However, most sufferers from TMDs are fairly young and otherwise healthy adults.

Diagnosis of TMDs

Over the years, various systems have been introduced to diagnose TMDs. Nowadays, the gold standard adopted by the international TMD research community is the Research Diagnostic Criteria (RDC/TMD) method. This standardised method of recording a patient's TMD history and examination considers two axes of diagnosis. Axis I is the physical diagnosis, which provides a description of the anatomical source of the patient's symptoms. Axis II provides a psychosocial diagnosis, but recording all the necessary information is time consuming and unlikely to be helpful in dental practice. Clinicians must, however, always bear in mind the psychosocial aspects of TMDs, recognising that if a patient appears depressed this may be a reaction to their jaw pain, not necessarily a cause of it.

The criteria to formulate the Axis I diagnosis are quite complex and aimed at research, but the simplicity of the final diagnosis into one of three categories is clinically extremely useful. The three diagnoses are:
• **Group I:** muscle (myofascial pain) characterised by muscle tenderness on palpation (see DVD video J).
• **Group II:** disc displacements with and without reduction (Figs 7-1 and 7-2) characterised by clicking (with reduction) and locking (without reduction).
• **Group III:** TMJ pain and degeneration:
  – arthralgia, characterised by local TMJ tenderness
  – arthrosis, characterised by crepitus
  – arthritis, characterised by crepitus and local TMJ tenderness.

Diagnoses from two or even all three of these main groups can occur together. The patient featured in the DVD video had TMJ tenderness on palpation, muscle tenderness in five locations, no limitation of jaw opening and an intermittent click on protrusion. The patient was suffering from myofascial pain. Although there was a click, it was non-reproducible and in all probability did not represent disc displacement with reduction. In relation to Group III, the patient had arthralgia (pain from the joint) but there were no clinical signs of arthrosis or arthritis. Therefore, in summary, the patient was diagnosed as having myofascial pain and arthralgia of the right TMJ.

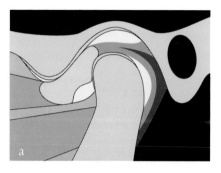
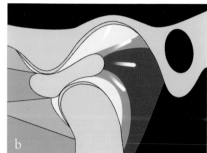
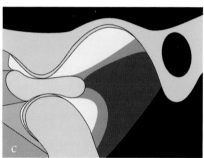

Fig 7-1 Disc displacement with reduction. (a) Disc displaced anteriorly or medially or both when in ICP. (b) On opening, the disc clicks back into place. (c) The disc remains in place until maximum opening but slips off the condyle again during closing.

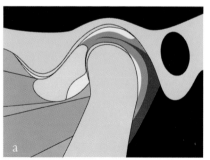
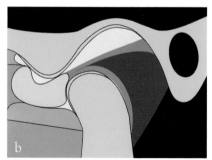

Fig 7-2 Disc displacement without reduction. (a) Disc displaced anteriorly or medially or both when in ICP. On opening, the disc does not go back into place but blocks condylar movement. (b) Maximum opening is often restricted, especially during the acute phase. The trapped disc may also cause mandibular deviation to the affected side.

Forms adapted to simplify the RDC for routine clinical care are available at *www.ncl.ac.uk/dental/AppliedOcclusion/*. These are recommended as a guideline for examination and diagnosis prior to undertaking complex and expensive treatment in cases in which there is any history of TMD.

Screening for TMD in Patients with Extensive Restorative Treatment Needs

Occlusal reorganisations and rehabilitations are often demanding and expensive courses of treatment. It is important therefore to know before you start treatment whether a patient has an underlying TMD. Furthermore, patients in need of extensive restoration are likely to undergo a number of occlusal changes during treatment; so if they are predisposed to TMD, great care must be taken. Screening for a history of TMD is, as a consequence, a wise precaution. Telltale signs include:

- clicking
- locking
- stiffness in the jaw muscles and joints, especially on waking
- difficulty with eating and jaw opening.

Unless the patient has a history of TMD, a full examination (as described in the DVD) would be excessive. A pragmatic alternative in patients without a history of TMD is to restrict the screening examination simply to muscle and joint palpation (checking for tenderness and joint sounds, as shown in the DVD) and to measuring for any signs of restricted jaw opening (Fig 7-3). If during the examination there are positive signs of TMD, the forms described in the previous section are helpful in making a simplified RDC physical diagnosis.

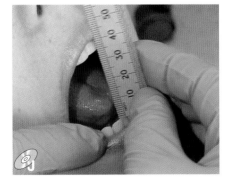

Fig 7-3 As part of screening for TMD, measure pain-free interincisal opening; <40 mm (including overbite) suggests limitation.

Obviously, telling the patient about the diagnosis is an important part of the process. Where there are signs of TMD, there is a decision to be made about whether you intend to treat the jaw problem before embarking on the restorative work, or whether you simply intend to note the problem and try to avoid aggravating it. Where symptoms are minor, for example a symptomless click, carrying out restorative work is often quite reasonable, particularly if occlusal disruption can be avoided. Incidentally, a mouth prop can be useful in some TMD patients to reduce discomfort associated with protracted periods of mouth opening.

Where there are greater problems, such as patients complaining of persistent facial pain, it is important to bear in mind that TMDs are not the only cause of non-dentally related pain. If diagnosis is in doubt, seek appropriate specialist advice, either before providing TMD treatment or, should a patient fail to respond, within two to three months of conservative management. The simple message here is to be cautious when extensive restorative treatment is planned for patients with facial or temporomandibular pain.

Occlusion as a Cause of TMDs

This has been the source of a great deal of heated discussion. Let us consider the evidence, or rather the lack of evidence, linking occlusion and TMDs. A large proportion of people have less than ideal occlusions – with missing teeth, interferences and deflective contacts – and do not suffer the slightest problem with their masticatory system. It is true that TMD patients may have a slightly greater prevalence of certain occlusal abnormalities than symptomless controls – including anterior open bite, a large overjet, multiple missing teeth, a slide from retruded contact position to intercuspal position (RCP–ICP slide) of >2 mm and unilateral posterior cross bite – but this is hardly proof of causation, and some of these occlusal features may have resulted from the TMD rather than have caused it.

If occlusal problems were the principal cause of TMDs, we would expect to find that occlusal adjustments and splints would offer significantly better treatment results than other forms of treatment across the spectrum of TMD sufferers. Recent systematic reviews suggest that the evidence for occlusal adjustment being more effective than placebo treatments is equivocal. They have shown little difference in effectiveness between splints with occlusal surfaces and those without – sometimes referred to as "placebo splints". Furthermore, there is no evidence that prophylactic occlusal adjustment can prevent the future onset of TMDs.

At a clinical level there is a danger of applying the findings of broad-brush reviews to a complex and multifactorial condition. This approach cannot adequately take into account the possibility that for a small but significant proportion of the TMD population there may actually be a meaningful occlusal element to the problem. Occlusally related treatments cannot be recommended for all patients, but there are, when carefully carried out within the operator's expertise, a small minority of patients for whom they are invaluable. The identification of patients in whom occlusal adjustments may be appropriate is considered later.

Treatment of TMDs

It would be inappropriate to attempt to cover TMD management comprehensively in this book. Suffice it to say that best practice is to provide an accurate diagnosis and then, wherever possible, reversible treatment in the first instance, namely:

- counselling
- self-help
- physiotherapy and jaw exercises
- analgesics
- occlusal splints.

Good communication is critical for the first two approaches.

Occlusal Splints

Occlusal splints are removable appliances, usually made of acrylic, which are fitted to the teeth of either jaw. They can be very effective as part of an overall management package.

Partial-coverage Splints

Partial-coverage splints are not recommended, as they can result in unwanted tooth movements and occlusal changes (Fig 7-4). Splints covering only the occlusal surfaces of the posterior teeth appear especially damaging in this respect, although intrusion and overeruption can occur with longer term wear of the variety of small anterior splints now commercially available, for example the NTI-TSS (Fig 7-5). These splints have a similar design to the Lucia jig, which can be indispensable for stabilising centric relation prior to registration. The construction of a Lucia jig is shown in the jaw registration DVD video (M) (see Section 8-4). Because of the risk of tooth movement and increased tooth mobility, some authorities utterly deprecate the use of

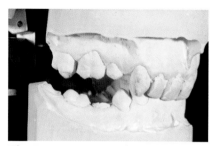

Fig 7-4 Severe tooth intrusion and overeruption associated with a posterior partial-coverage splint.

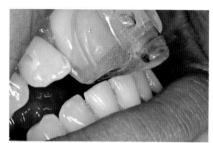

Fig 7-5 The NTI-TSS splint is a small partial-coverage splint, which should be worn intermittently and not for long periods to prevent unwanted tooth movement.

such splints in TMD management. The splints can, however, occasionally be useful in patients with myofascial pain and headaches associated with nocturnal parafunctional activity who seem unable to tolerate larger full-coverage splints. Provided they are only used for night wear, the risks of long-term occlusal changes should be minimised.

Soft Splints

Soft splints produced from heat- and vacuum-formed vinyl are frequently prescribed. These are generally useful as part of an overall TMD treatment package, though the mechanism of action is unclear. Some patients report that soft splints make their discomfort worse, possibly through clenching on the resilient surface. In addition, they are of limited value in patients having problems with mandibular alignment associated with deflective contacts and interferences. In both of these situations, a stabilisation splint is a better option.

Stabilisation Splints

Although clinical research reports little difference in TMD treatment outcomes between different splint designs, clinical experience suggests that a carefully adjusted stabilisation splint (Fig 7-6) can be helpful, particularly in those patients whose disrupted occlusion may have precipitated or perpetuated their condition, either through increased muscle activity or adverse posture, creating stresses and instability in the TMJs. The sorts of patients for whom this may be helpful are, for example, those with a substantial asymmetric RCP–ICP slide. This results in one or both mandibular condyles being distracted from the fossae. In itself this is not normally serious, but if combined with other

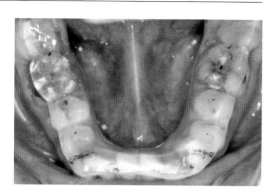

Fig 7-6 Stabilisation splints can be made for the lower or upper jaw. They provide full coverage, therefore preventing unwanted tooth movement.

factors, for example a parafunctional clenching habit, then it is perhaps not surprising that the joint and muscles may start to ache. It is like going for a long run in odd shoes or cycling a long distance on bent pedals! At other times, it is more difficult to predict an underlying occlusal problem, which may only show itself – perhaps as a small but irritating interference – after the splint has allowed the mandible to find a position of musculoskeletal stability and neuromuscular balance.

The design of stabilisation splints is considered further in Chapter 8. Such splints are an important element of the management armamentarium. The basic principle in managing TMDs is to cover the cusps and provide a flat surface, allowing the mandible to find a comfortable position without deflective contacts. In this way the condyles are able to rest fully in the glenoid fossae in the hinge axis. The splint is also usually designed to provide canine guidance and posterior disclusion on lateral excursions, meaning that all aspects of the occlusion are controlled and predictable.

Particularly where there is derangement within the joint or where the muscles are tense, dentists need to carry out adjustments not only when fitting a stabilisation splint but also on review. We suggest the following treatment regimen:
1. Schedule the first review appointment after one or two weeks to check the splint with shim stock and articulating paper for even occlusion with smooth but shallow anterior guidance.
2. Advise the patient to wear the splint as much as possible to reduce the amount of natural tooth contact. In this way, problems with mandibular alignment are most easily rectified, though there are practical limitations for the patient if day wear will interfere with normal activities.

3. Continue with two-week reviews and adjustments until the splint has a stable occlusion. Most patients reach stability very quickly with minimal follow-up adjustment, although for others it can take several months and the adjustment is trickier.

As regards reducing pain intensity, this takes on average three months to reach a plateau, although response is usually faster at the beginning of treatment. Patients also need to know that clicking is difficult to eliminate, but that it can usually be made less intense and more comfortable.

Anterior Positioning Splints

These splints (Fig 7-7a,b) are rather specialist and are used to try to "recapture" an anteriorly displaced disc; in other words, we use it for patients who have a troublesome, reproducible TMJ click on either opening or closing, or both. A reasonable clinical test is to get the patient to protrude their mandible, which

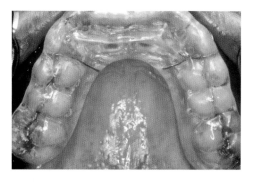

Fig 7-7a The anterior positioning appliance is also a full-coverage splint sometimes used to treat clicking.

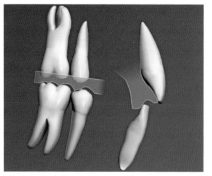
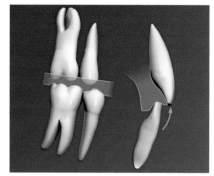

Fig 7-7b The ramps on the splint act to hold the mandible downwards and forwards in an attempt to "recapture" a displaced disk.

should eliminate the click and make the affected joint feel more comfortable. Considering the number of people with clicking jaws, we use this splint design only rarely, and we always bear in mind the possibility that long-term use can result in major occlusal disruption. This can take the form of a posterior open bite, possibly resulting from remodelling within the TMJs. We therefore advise patients to wean themselves off the splint after three months.

Dentists sometimes adjust the patient's occlusion after splint treatment, but for most patients this is unnecessary overtreatment. The following section considers the rationale for occlusal adjustment in TMD patients.

Occlusal Adjustment

Initial Adjustment
For most TMD patients occlusal adjustment is neither desirable nor helpful as a first line of treatment, and an imprecise adjustment can be positively harmful. However, there are a few situations where occlusal adjustment may form part of primary treatment to eliminate deflective contacts or interferences:

- associated with an overerupted and unopposed wisdom tooth (Fig 7-8); in this case the tooth is often best removed, as further overeruption will exacerbate occlusal instability
- associated with a recently placed restoration apparently responsible for the onset of TMD
- where a deflective contact is so large that splint treatment is not feasible without some adjustment.

Where the placement of multiple restorations has caused occlusal disharmony and associated TMD, a period of splint treatment is often necessary to stabilise the jaws prior to occlusal adjustment.

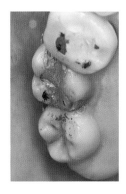

Fig 7-8 An overerupted maxillary wisdom tooth causing an unstable deflective contact (marked facet on mesio-lingual cusp). To avoid problems when fitting a full-coverage splint, we often extract such teeth first and review. Symptoms sometimes resolve without any further treatment, but this cannot be guaranteed.

Adjustment Following Splint Treatment

Following stabilisation splint treatment it may be worth considering the need for occlusal adjustment when:

- on removing the splint the patient notices a return of symptoms, which is relieved on replacing the splint
- teeth affected by occlusal discrepancies need to be restored in any case
- teeth affected by occlusal discrepancies show signs of damage or trauma from the occlusion.

Given the lack of a strong association between occlusal factors and TMDs, dentists should always be able to justify the prescription of an occlusal adjustment from either a restorative or a functional aspect. The same advice applies to the replacement of missing teeth.

Conclusions

- Signs and symptoms of TMD are seen commonly in the general population, but only a small proportion (2–7%) needs treatment.
- Patients needing restorative work should be screened for underlying TMDs to avoid inadvertently precipitating further problems during treatment.
- Remember that TMD may occasionally present as part of a systemic condition (fibromyalgia, rheumatoid arthritis, systemic joint laxity).
- For most TMD patients the occlusion appears of little relevance, although in a small but significant proportion there may be a meaningful occlusal element.
- Dentists should be able to diagnose accurately the physical signs of TMDs.
- Occlusal treatment is but one facet of TMD management and with few exceptions should be reversible.

Further Reading

De Boever JA, Carlsson GE, Klineberg IJ. Need for occlusal therapy and prosthodontic treatment in the management of temporomandibular disorders. Part I: Occlusal interferences and occlusal adjustment. J Oral Rehabil 2000;27(5):367–379.

De Boever JA, Carlsson GE, Klineberg IJ. Need for occlusal therapy and prosthodontic treatment in the management of temporomandibular disorders. Part II: Tooth loss and prosthodontic treatment. J Oral Rehabil 2000;27(8):647–659.

Diatchenko L, Slade GD, Nackley AG, et al. Genetic basis for individual variations in pain perception and the development of a chronic pain condition. Hum Mol Genet 2005;14(1):135–143.

Dworkin SF, LeResche L. Research diagnostic criteria for temporomandibular disorders: review, criteria, examinations and specifications, critique. J Craniomandib Disord 1992;6(4):301–355.

Forssell H, Kalso E. Application of principles of evidence-based medicine to occlusal treatment for temporomandibular disorders: are there lessons to be learned? J Orofac Pain 2004;18(1):9–22; discussion 23–32.

Okeson JP. Management of Temporomandibular Disorders. 6th edn. St. Louis: Elsevier, Mosby, 2008.

Pullinger AG, Seligman DA, Gornbein JA. A multiple logistic regression analysis of the risk and relative odds of temporomandibular disorders as a function of common occlusal features. J Dent Res 1993;72(6):968–979.

Wassell RW, Adams N, Kelly PJ. The treatment of temporomandibular disorders with stabilizing splints in general dental practice: one-year follow-up. J Am Dent Assoc 2006;137(8):1089–1098.

Chapter 8
Occlusal Techniques

Introduction

In the preceding chapters, we have explored many of the concepts that link occlusion and restorative dentistry. The aim of this chapter is to consider the techniques used routinely to treat occlusally related problems or to plan and provide restorations requiring occlusal control. Practical courses are the best way to learn some of the key techniques, but the text and the DVD are intended to provide considerable insight to allow the reader to learn them in a clinical setting.

There are 12 sections in this chapter. The sections with the DVD logo have an associated video showing the relevant clinical and laboratory stages for a patient diagnosed with a functional occlusal problem. It is worth re-emphasising the message in the introduction of this book that these stages are common to many occlusal diagnoses and treatments.

8-1 OCCLUSAL EXAMINATION

A detailed occlusal examination of patients presenting with problems such as unexplained pain, wear, fracture, drifting and mobility (see Chapter 2) is an integral, invaluable part of the dental examination. A detailed occlusal examination is essential when planning any major restorative work to determine, for example, whether this should be provided as a conformative or reorganised procedure and to consider whether any occlusal adjustments are needed before providing definitive restorations (see Chapter 3). The clinical technique for carrying out a full occlusal examination is shown on the DVD.

Do I Need to Do a Full Occlusal Examination?

The answer in most cases is no. The extent of the examination will vary from patient to patient. It is possible to identify isolated occlusal problems without systematically following the procedure shown in the video, but this requires intuition and experience. A systematic approach is usually needed to resolve more complex problems. It is worth practising all parts of the examination when the opportunity arises, particularly techniques such as identifying guidance teeth and finding the hinge axis, so that they become second nature.

Some find it helpful to use a structured record form, but, once you are familiar with carrying out an occlusal examination, the relevant findings can be recorded as shown in Table 8-1.

"Good" and "Bad" Contacts

In essence, the occlusal examination allows important tooth contacts to be identified. There are "good" contacts, which support the occlusion and guide jaw movement, and "bad" contacts, which deflect jaw movement during closure or interfere with excursions. It is also important to identify those contacts which would otherwise be good, but which occur on teeth that are heavily restored and poorly equipped to handle the loads that result from guidance or parafunction.

Although most people are not troubled by deflective contacts and interferences, in some patients they are associated with problems such as pain, fracture, mobility and wear. Furthermore, the inadvertent removal of contacts during tooth preparation can give rise to unwanted changes in jaw position and loss of occlusal space, as described in Chapter 3. It is sensible to know in advance of preparing a tooth whether it includes a holding or guidance contact which needs to be incorporated in the restoration. A deflective contact or interference, however, can be eliminated before preparing the tooth, and so avoid reproducing it in the restoration. Detecting such contacts can be quickly and easily achieved with a systematic examination.

Deflective contacts and interferences may occur developmentally, but are often the result of tooth movements caused by extractions, poorly contoured restorations, periodontal disease, periapical inflammation and tooth wear. More unusual causes of deflective contacts and interferences include jaw fracture and tooth movements occurring during pregnancy (Fig 8-1). Whatever the cause, the principles of examining and adjusting the occlusion are the same.

Screening for Parafunction

It is always worth knowing if the patient is a bruxist, as this will help in both the diagnosis of problems of excessive occlusal loading (see Chapter 3) and the prescription of suitably robust restorations. Parafunction is often episodic, and so the detection of faceting and vertical microfractures does not mean that bruxism is active at that time. Clinical indicators of active parafunction include fremitus, tooth tenderness and ridging of the sides of the tongue or cheeks at the level of the occlusal plane.

Table 8-1 **An ordered occlusal examination: simply list relevant clinical findings against each component**

Component of examination	What to look for
Separate arches	• Signs of occlusal overload: obvious facets, vertical enamel fractures, abfraction • Signs of occlusal instability: drifting and mobility not explained by periodontal disease
Intercuspal position (ICP)	• Assess posterior support: pairs of teeth on each side holding shim stock • Appearance of occlusal markings: small and discrete or broad and rubbing – see below • Assess potential for anterior guidance: horizontal and vertical overlap, occlusal plane
Retruded contact position (RCP)	• Identify teeth providing RCP contact – see below • Does the retruded contact appear to be associated with occlusal problems? • Is the contact likely to be removed during tooth preparation for restorations?
RCP–ICP slide	• Assess the slide both quantitatively and qualitatively – see below • Look for evidence of an anterior thrust: e.g. localised wear on palatal aspects of upper anterior teeth and fremitus – see below
Right lateral excursion (RLE)	• Note the guidance teeth and interferences on the working and non-working sides
Left lateral excursion (LLE)	• As for RLE
Protrusion	• Note the guidance teeth: interferences are usually on the posterior teeth
Loss of vertical dimension	• Where indicated, measure occlusal and rest vertical dimensions • Also take into account facial profile, need for interocclusal space and aesthetic requirements

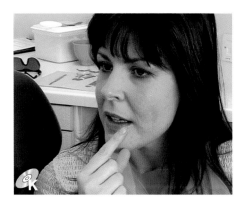

Fig 8-1 The patient shown on the DVD reported a clear history of occlusal changes during pregnancy which, despite an excellent periodontal condition, had not resolved over a year later.

Screening for Temporomandibular Disorders

As discussed in Chapter 7, it is also good practice to check all patients for signs and symptoms of temporomandibular disorders (TMDs), particularly those patients requiring extensive restorations. Screening for a history of a painful or clicking jaw, muscle and/or temporomandibular joint (TMJ) tenderness on examination, significant joint sounds (bearing in mind that mild clicking is very common) and limitation of jaw movement is appropriate for all patients.

Reserve the full TMD examination (shown in DVD video J) for patients who have a significant problem requiring more detailed diagnosis. A screening check can be combined with a brief occlusal examination.

Performing the Examination

The following sections are intended to be used in conjunction with Table 8-1 and the relevant video clips on the DVD.

What Instruments Do I Need?
Set up an examination tray (Fig 8-2) with thin articulating foils (< 20 μm thick) and shim stock. The foils are much easier to use if held in Miller's forceps to stop them crumpling. Use one colour, for example black, for ICP marks and another, for example red, for excursive marks. Shim stock is a 10 μm-thick Mylar film and is held in mosquito forceps. It is used as a feeler gauge between occluding teeth. The extent of posterior contact can be quantified as the number of pairs of posterior teeth holding the shim. Some way of measuring the vertical dimension, such as a Willis gauge, may also be useful.

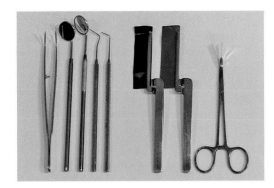

Fig 8-2 Examination tray for occlusal examination, with Miller's forceps holding black and red articulating foil and mosquito forceps holding shim stock.

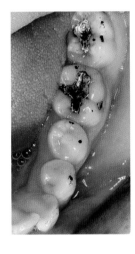

Fig 8-3 ICP contacts are ideally small and discrete.

8-4 ICP contacts that are broad and rubbing are sometimes associated with underlying occlusal problems.

What Should ICP Occlusal Contacts Look Like?

Occlusal contacts do not always mark well with thin occlusal marking foils, particularly if the teeth are wet. Sometimes the situation can be improved by first marking the teeth with a thicker paper, which leaves a broad smudge of colour against which the contrasting colour of the finer foil can be seen. The best way of ensuring you can see contacts is by making the teeth dry.

In the young, ICP contacts should ideally be small and discrete, with multiple contacts on each tooth providing occlusal stability (Fig 8-3). ICP contacts that are broad and rubbing, as seen in the patient in the DVD (Fig 8-4), can signify occlusal instability when associated with functional disturbances. Bear in mind, however, that the area of contacts can also increase with normal levels of wear.

91

Do ICP Tooth Relationships Potentially Affect Anterior Guidance?

Before looking at mandibular excursions, the ICP can tell you quite a lot about guidance. If there is little or no vertical overlap of incisors or canines, the capacity of these teeth to guide jaw movement, with the disclusion of the posterior teeth, will be limited or non-existent. Similarly, if the overbite is incomplete, there may be a considerable delay during excursions before the anterior teeth come into contact.

Rather more difficult to comprehend is the effect of the occlusal plane. On the one hand, a flat occlusal plane with a shallow angle to the horizontal plane – the patient's Frankfort plane – will dispose to posterior disclusion. On the other hand, a curved occlusal plane, or one with a steep angle to the horizontal, will dispose to clashing of posterior teeth. Cross-bites and scissor bites – the upper teeth occluding buccal to the lower teeth – often cause interferences or deflective contacts.

How Do I Assess the RCP–ICP Slide?

This is one of the most important skills to learn for assessing the occlusion. It is not difficult, but it only comes with practice. Using bimanual manipulation, with the patient completely relaxed and preferably supine, guide the patient into RCP (Fig 8-5a,b).

Ask the patient to point to the contacting teeth and feel how the mandible slides into ICP. Qualitatively, the slide will either be present or absent, smooth or rough, small or large. Quantitatively, estimate how far the mandible deviates

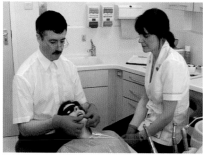

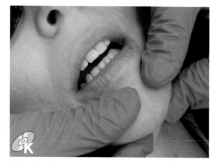

Fig 8-5a Bimanual manipulation is used to seat the condyles in centric relation to examine the retruded contact and the RCP–ICP slide.

Fig 8-5b Manipulation should take place with the patient supine and teeth only slightly separated.

forwards or laterally by looking at the relationship between the upper and lower incisors during the slide. Chapter 3 and the DVD illustrate how to do this, looking both from in front and from the side of the patient.

How Do I Detect Fremitus?

Look out for an anterior thrust associated with a deflective RCP–ICP slide. Often, anterior teeth affected by an anterior thrust will exhibit fremitus, as do some teeth involved in guidance. You can easily detect fremitus as palpable vibration by placing your index finger on each of the teeth in turn and asking the patient to tap together. With marked fremitus, the vibrations will be clearly visible. The anterior thrust may also be associated with specific problems with the upper anterior teeth, such as localised palatal wear, damage to restorations or incisor drifting.

What Do I Need To Look for with Excursive Movements?

The important thing is to identify which teeth guide movement and which teeth interfere with it. Excursive contacts, when marked with foil, should appear smooth and unbroken. An irregular, broken or dog-legged appearance suggests an interference, either on the tooth itself or on a tooth distant to it (Fig 8-6a,b).

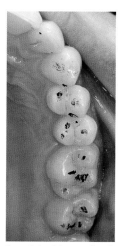

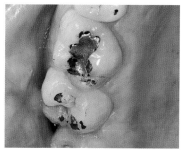

Fig 8-6a Markings for left lateral excursion showing poorly defined guidance on the canine. The difficulty the patient had in making this movement suggested the heavier red marks on the premolars were interferences.

Fig 8-6b There were also non-working-side interferences (again marked in red) on the upper right first and second molars.

In simple terms, the jaws and TMJs comprise a lever system. Forces applied to the teeth by the masticatory muscles diminish as you move anteriorly. Hence, anterior teeth are better positioned than posterior teeth to accept the non-axial forces associated with excursive loading of the mandible. Nevertheless, posterior teeth are often involved in guiding jaw movements. Provided these contacts are in harmony, the system works well.

Sometimes, as shown in the DVD (animation I) and discussed in more detail in Chapter 3, posterior contacts can act as pivots or fulcrums. In making assessments about whether and how such pivots may need to be managed, mounted casts usefully supplement the clinical occlusal examination.

When Do I Need to Assess Vertical Dimension?
The simple answer is, when you might be thinking about changing it. In practice this will be for very few patients. These tend to be patients who appear to have lost occlusal vertical dimension (OVD), either with excessive wear or tooth loss, and where an increase in OVD, and therefore an occlusal reorganisation, is planned. Excessive tooth wear is often compensated for by dentoalveolar extrusion. Even where there is considerable wear, the freeway space may be "normal", but that does not preclude a change (see Chapter 4).

The usual procedure is to measure the OVD and resting vertical dimension with a Willis gauge. Subtracting one from the other gives the freeway space. With the patient sitting upright, the normal range of freeway space is 2–4 mm. This is notoriously imprecise because of its inherent variability and measurement inaccuracies, arising largely from compressibility of the soft tissues.

Do I Need Mounted Casts?
The answer to this is no, not for routine examinations. They can, however, be invaluable for planning treatment, communicating with the laboratory and explaining treatment to the patient. If you intend to perform irreversible changes to the occlusion as part of a restorative treatment plan, mounted casts are indispensable, both as a baseline record and in the planning of occlusal alterations. Changes to the occlusion often involve trial adjustments and diagnostic waxing (see Sections 8-7 and 8-8). Two sets of casts are therefore recommended, so that one set can be kept unchanged.

8-2 Accurate Alginate Impressions

Many dentists treat alginate as a humble and somewhat inaccurate material. But accuracy is paramount when articulating diagnostic casts and when preparing opposing casts for indirect restorations. The opposing impression is often the last procedure following successful completion of preparation, temporisation and the working impression, and so it can end up as a bit of an afterthought. The implications of an inaccurate opposing impression are far from trivial. Precious time can be lost adjusting the occlusal surface of a crown because the opposing alginate impression was distorted or carelessly recorded, making for unnecessary expense, and the clinical outcome can be compromised. Simple quality control at this stage can save a lot of subsequent grief.

A high degree of accuracy can be achieved by avoiding common pitfalls and by being prepared to spend a few seconds checking the impression before sending it to the laboratory. Clearly, disinfection, bagging up to avoid drying out and ensuring alginates are cast within a few hours are essential measures.

The DVD shows a number of tips, including:
- the use of rim-lock trays (Fig 8-7)
- drying the teeth and smearing material on the occlusal surfaces prior to seating the tray to avoid occlusal air blows (Fig 8-8)
- pulling unset material over the heel of the tray with a mouth mirror to help keep the impression in the tray on removal from the mouth
- trimming the impression to allow inspection and reduce distortions prior to pouring up (Fig 8-9)
- careful inspection of the impression.

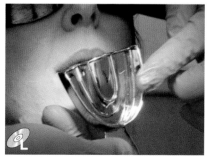

Fig 8-7 Rim-lock trays are a good option for alginate impressions.

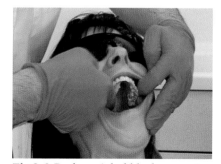

Fig 8-8 Reduce air bubbles by smearing alginate onto the occlusal surfaces.

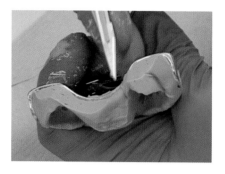

Fig 8-9 Always trim the heel and check the impression has not pulled away.

Perforated stock trays often come in a limited range of sizes and often do not fit well, sometimes failing to cover the most posterior teeth. It is not a problem to extend a stock tray – unless you choose to use wax. Unfortunately, wax distorts easily, and so distorts the alginate it is supposed to be supporting. A better option is to use impression compound (greenstick), which is rigid. The softened material is applied to the upper and lower surfaces of the tray heels and then teased out in sufficient thickness to include all the teeth in the tray. Perforated stock trays can occasionally cause problems when the alginate partly pulls out of the perforations on removal from the mouth. If you do not use adhesive with a perforated tray or you give insufficient time for the adhesive solvent to evaporate, the risk of this distortion is greatly increased. The rule is: use an adhesive and let it dry before the impression is taken.

Rim-lock trays are a good alternative to perforated trays. They come in a good range of sizes and can retain an alginate impression without the use of an adhesive. The disadvantages of rim-lock trays include ensuring their return from the laboratory and difficulties in cleaning prior to decontamination and sterilisation.

Although the cost of material is much higher, it is worth considering a fast-setting addition silicone as an alternative to alginate, particularly when multiple casts are required. Unlike alginate, silicone impressions can be re-poured without significant loss of accuracy. When taking impressions for study models in complex cases, this may prove to be cost effective. The use of a perforated tray is recommended for silicones, as silicone adhesives are more effective than those used for alginates. The set material is also more rigid and, therefore, more difficult to remove from the mouth.

8-3 INTERCUSPAL REGISTRATION

ICP or Centric Relation Registration?

In the previous section, consideration was given to the importance of accurate alginate impressions, both for diagnostic casts and for opposing casts when making indirect restorations. One of the greatest sources of confusion relates to what type of registration should be used to articulate sets of casts. Put very simply, ICP registration is used to construct restorations on working casts, while centric relation (CR) registration is for diagnosis and treatment planning. For any given case, you might start with casts mounted in CR and plan treatment on this basis. You would then decide to conform to what is there, in which case you use ICP records to make your restorations or to reorganise, creating a new ICP in CR.

This, of course, is not absolute. Casts mounted in ICP – even hand-held casts – might provide some useful diagnostic information, but remember they give no information on deflective contacts and, at best, limited information on guidance and excursive interferences. Furthermore, restorations may, on occasion, be made on casts mounted in CR.

Mounting Casts in ICP

The fundamental problem with any interocclusal record used to articulate casts is that there is a substantial risk of the record itself preventing the casts coming fully together. An intervening layer of registration material commonly creates the sort of occlusal error that one is trying to avoid. Often, the best occlusal record is no occlusal record at all. Where one is used, it should be as minimal as is required to locate the casts accurately.

Diagnostic casts are often held in ICP by hand. This is quick and often effective when the teeth locate in a stable position. This approach can, however, mislead diagnosis. Problems with hand-held casts occur when they cannot be easily and reliably located in a stable intercuspal relationship. The reasons may include:
- distorted casts – undetected impression distortion can result in normal looking casts
- blebs and faults on the occlusal surfaces
- a limited number and arrangement of teeth
- malocclusions, such as open bites (Fig 8-10) or cusp-to-cusp occlusion
- incorrect assumptions regarding the orientation of the occlusal plane.

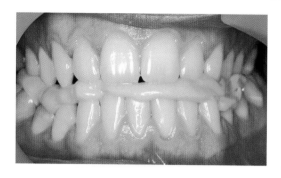

Fig 8-10 Silicone ICP record used for a patient with an anterior open bite – a rare case in which a full-arch record is justified.

All these factors can make it impossible to locate and record a reproducible, let alone relevant, position. In the event of an error, it may be necessary to start again, modify the casts to remove blebs or imperfections, or to use a different approach to registration to allow the casts to be mounted in an articulator. Articulator choice is covered in Section 8-6.

Working casts for indirect restorations are generally mounted in some form of articulator. An interocclusal record is often necessary to achieve this, but not always. The general principle is to limit, where possible, the ICP record to the preparations and the opposing teeth. In this way the unprepared teeth are not prevented from coming into contact by the record. This principle applies whatever material is used.

A full-arch record is almost never needed, perhaps only where there is an anterior open bite and the casts rock; but even then, trimmed localised records may be possible. Less is often more with ICP records.

Materials for ICP Records

The choice of materials for ICP registration is generally between:
• nothing at all
• silicone mousse
• wax sheet, horseshoe or section
• wax rims
• acrylic copings and stents.

A combination of materials is sometimes required, as indicated below.

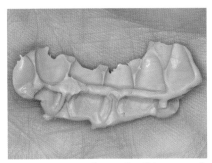 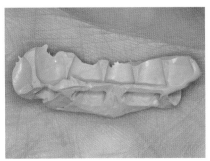

Fig 8-11a Superfluous detail in a record, including embrasures and gingival tissues, can prevent it seating on the casts.

Fig 8-11b Following disinfection, the record should be trimmed with a scalpel to leave only areas essential for location.

Silicone Mousse

The important thing to remember about this type of material is that it needs to be trimmed, whether it is being used as a sectional or full-arch registration (Fig 8-11a,b). Another important point is that a silicone mousse records surface detail very well, often better than the material used to record the impressions. In other words, the detail recorded by the mousse may prevent the two casts seating in the record. Without trimming, and sometimes even with trimming, the mounting will often feel springy when the registration is sandwiched between the casts. Simply squeezing the casts together with, for example, an elastic band is not the answer, as the material will deform under pressure, resulting in unpredictable occlusal changes. Usually, trimming the record with a scalpel will allow an accurate mounting. It is equally important that bubbles and blebs on the casts are removed.

Wax Sheet, Horseshoe or Section

A "wax bite" horseshoe or sheet is often used as an intercuspal record. Unlike silicone mousse materials, waxes are not dimensionally stable and are very easily deformed in transit to the laboratory. As with silicone mousse materials, pressing casts into a wax record will result in an incorrect articulation. Wax is occasionally used for sectional ICP records (Fig 8-12).

With this technique, distortion is minimised as there is no cross-arch recording and the record is small enough to minimise the risk of it not seating. The use of a full-arch wax bite is rarely indicated as an intercuspal record as the risk of introducing an error in articulation is considerable.

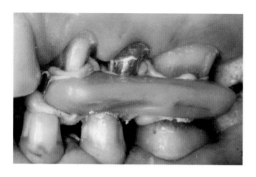

Fig 8-12 A localised wax and registration paste record offers the advantage of keeping unprepared teeth in contact. Again, trim for proper seating on casts.

Waxes are available in various consistencies, ranging from the comparatively soft, through pink modelling wax to hard wax. There is little clinical evidence to support the use of any particular wax.

Wax Rims

Although silicone mousse registrations are surprisingly versatile, large edentulous areas may make it difficult to obtain a stable mounting without using wax occlusal registration rims, as one would use for partial denture construction. Wax rims are, however, supported only by soft tissues, so when patients bite onto a wax rim the baseplate is displaced into the soft tissues. As dental stone is not compressible like mucosa, this results in an inaccurate registration when the rim is transferred onto the cast. To minimise this, trim away the occlusal indentations in the rim until there is firm contact on the teeth and only light contact on the rim, so that it is sitting passively on the mucosa. Then record ICP with a thin layer of registration paste or silicone mousse placed on top of the rim; being fluid, these materials do not displace the rim into the mucosa.

Bear in mind that a baseplate made on the cast from one impression cannot reliably be transferred to a cast poured from another – there are always differences between casts recorded by multiple impressions. If a wax occlusal rim is needed, it is best made on the working cast, not transferred from study models.

Increasing Vertical Dimension, Acrylic Copings and Stents

When a registration is used in the construction of definitive restorations at an increased vertical dimension, the mandibular position is best stabilised during the procedure by using one or more provisional restorations made at the desired dimension. Of course, in such cases the new ICP is also in CR.

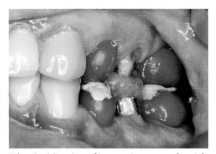 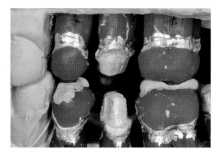

Fig 8-13a Acrylic copings used with registration paste for a posterior reconstruction.

Fig 8-13b Casts with silver dies mounted.

Some operators prefer to use acrylic copings to record ICP when managing more extensive cases (Fig 8-13), particularly where opposing arches are being restored simultaneously. These techniques are more involved, but in extensive cases the accuracy they allow can be invaluable. Copings are made either on silver dies or duplicate stone dies to prevent damage to the originals. The advantage is that mounting accuracy can be checked on the articulator using shim stock between both opposing copings and unprepared teeth. Rather than linking opposing copings together, the upper copings are made with a rounded occlusal excrescence, which is coated in petroleum jelly. This excrescence indents into registration material placed on the occlusal surface of the lower coping. Traditionally, self-cured acrylic is used as the registration material, but registration paste can be used. This has the advantages of not setting as quickly or undergoing polymerisation shrinkage, as occurs with acrylic. The paste can be made to stick to the coping by first applying a coat of dental varnish.

As shown in Fig 8-14, some configurations of teeth can be difficult to register, particularly when teeth oppose on edentulous space. One solution is to

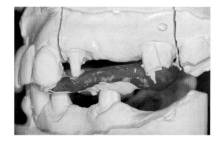

Fig 8-14 "Battlement occlusion" causes difficulty in having no directly opposing teeth for registration. A rigid acrylic stent provides greater reliability than wax rims.

101

construct an acrylic stent or bar; this acts as a rigid vehicle to carry registration material, thereby avoiding the less reliable wax occlusal rims. In situations where you are doubtful about the accuracy of a registration it is worth having a metal try-in, which can be used as a form of registration coping to check and, if necessary, remount before the porcelain is applied.

Checking the Registration

A written record of the existing intercuspal contacts can be helpful to the technician to ensure that casts are correctly mounted. Some operators draw a diagram of the pattern of occlusal contacts marked with articulating foil. A simpler alternative is to record pairs of teeth that resist the removal of shim stock.

8-4 CENTRIC RELATION REGISTRATION

Why Choose CR?

Mounting casts in ICP is common practice. As discussed in the previous section, this is the position used typically for the construction of restorations conforming to an existing occlusion. Casts mounted in ICP can be used for diagnosis, but for the reasons mentioned previously they are wholly inadequate in more extensive cases. In these situations it is necessary to consider occlusal contacts relative to CR. Concerning the planning and construction of restorations, there are two specific situations where you might choose to mount casts in CR:

• Diagnostic casts where you plan either to adjust or to reorganise the occlusion, including any case where you are planning to change the vertical dimension.

• Working casts where the occlusion is being reorganised using indirect restorations to establish a new ICP in CR. This may occur when adhesively retained restorations are used to increase vertical dimension, providing the basis of a new ICP at an early stage of reorganisation (see Chapter 4). The new ICP is sometimes termed "centric occlusion", which is defined as the occlusion that occurs in CR.

In such circumstances, the casts must be mounted to provide an accurate simulation of mandibular movement around CR, particularly during opening and closing. This involves mounting the upper cast on an appropriate articulator (see Section 8-6) using a facebow (see Section 8-5) and then mounting the lower cast with a CR registration.

As with an ICP record, obtaining accuracy to within a few micrometres is necessary if you are to make the most of the technology you are using.

What Techniques Are Available?

Being able to find the hinge axis and then record it is an essential skill in restorative dentistry. This gets much easier with practise. If finding the hinge axis is something you find difficult, then you are not alone. It is something you can practise on any patient. Once you have mastered the technique, it becomes a matter of routine.

The simplest and most frequently used technique involves bimanual manipulation to locate the patient's condyles in CR (Fig 8-15) and then taking

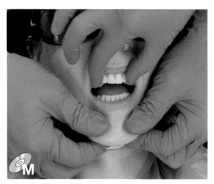

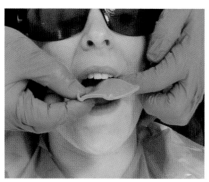

Fig 8-15 The nurse holds the wax record while the dentist uses bimanual manipulation to seat the condyles fully in their fossae.

Fig 8-16 Remove the record, chill under cold water, replace and check the teeth close cleanly into the indentations. This gives an indication of reproducibility.

a hard wax record, as shown in detail on the DVD. With practice, this approach works very well for most patients. It has the advantage that you can readily re-manipulate the jaw to assess whether the teeth re-engage cleanly into the indentations (Fig 8-16).

However, this technique is useless in cases in which a patient has mobile teeth, which will displace on closing into the viscous wax. In such circumstance it is better to use a low-viscosity material, such as a silicone registration mousse, or a traditional zinc-oxide eugenol registration paste carried on a gauze frame. The DVD shows how a silicone mousse record can be made.

When using a fluid material, a stable anterior stop is imperative for the mandibular incisors to rest against (Fig 8-17a,b). Otherwise, it is impossible to hold the mandible steady while the material sets, and the patient invariably slips back into ICP. For this purpose, it is helpful to use a Lucia jig at the selected vertical dimension, as described below.

What About Patients Who Are Difficult to Manipulate?

The ability to find the hinge axis depends as much on your own demeanour as on the cooperation of the patient. The patient needs to relax, and so does the dentist. Having the patient supine is helpful, as is a calm voice – which you must maintain no matter how frustrated you may have become trying to find CR.

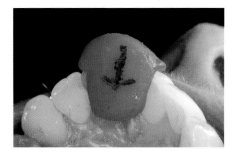

Fig 8-17a Lucia jig showing the arrowhead tracing for a single lower incisor making lateral and protrusive excursions.

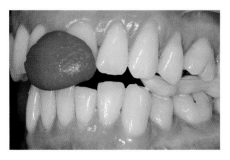

Fig 8-17b Silicone mousse used for jaw registration while the Lucia jig stabilises the jaw in CR. If there is sufficient space, syringe the mousse from the buccal aspects. Alternatively, syringe the mousse onto the occlusal surfaces of the lower arch and manipulate the patient into CR.

Nevertheless, some patients are difficult to manipulate. You can help such patients relax their mandible during jaw registration by preventing their teeth from closing into ICP for a few minutes by placing either a cotton wool roll or a tongue spatula between the incisors. Alternatively, you can use a slightly more sophisticated approach by forming a simple, flat, anterior jig made of self-cured acrylic – a Lucia jig. The key to success with a Lucia jig is to ensure that the occluding portion lies flat against no more than two incisors. Any indentations in the surface of the jig will only serve to guide the patient repeatedly back to an incorrect position. In essence, the jig, cotton wool roll or tongue spatula encourages the neuromuscular system to "forget" the ICP, the memory of which is reinforced by proprioceptive feedback every time the patient swallows.

Usually, simple techniques for separating the teeth are sufficient to allow successful bimanual manipulation. Indeed, some patients will experience "neuromuscular release", whereby the mandible, previously affected by muscle splinting, suddenly becomes easy to manipulate. Nevertheless, in a small minority of patients, the muscle splinting consistently returns the teeth to ICP and the mandible remains extremely difficult to manipulate. For such patients you may need to consider, as a last resort, making them an occlusal stabilisation splint to condition the masticatory system before recording CR (see Section 8-10). Paradoxically, a CR registration is normally used for the construction of stabilisation splints, which implies that a certain amount of splint adjustment may be needed after fitting.

Electrical stimulation may be used in an attempt to condition the masticatory muscles prior to recording CR, together with electromyographic instrumentation to determine lack of muscle splinting. At the present time there is no strong evidence base to support such an approach.

How Can You Check a CR Registration?

The easiest way to check a CR registration, as shown on the DVD, is to inspect the mounted casts to see if they simulate the retruded contact and then the RCP–ICP slide. Of course you will need to lift, or possibly remove, the pin in the articulator to do this. Identifying which teeth make retruded contact is easy on an articulator, but it takes practice to determine if the RCP–ICP slide is similar to that in the patient. If the casts cannot be fully interdigitated in ICP, this may reflect a registration inaccuracy or a limitation in the function of the articulator.

Some articulator manufacturers supply devices to check the reproducibility of multiple CR registrations, for example the Denar Vericheck. This resembles an articulator, but with its condylar and fossa elements replaced by styli and paper flags. It requires three separate jaw registrations. Each registration is placed in turn between the casts mounted on the instrument and four styli marks are made – two horizontal and two vertical – representing a notional terminal hinge axis. If the styli marks from all three registrations correspond, you can be confident about the registration. If the marks do not correspond, the registration with the most superior/posterior position of the hinge axis is taken as the best attempt – but bear in mind it may still be incorrect. These are useful teaching and research instruments, but they find limited application in clinical practice.

8-5 FACEBOW RECORD

As shown on the DVD, a facebow record takes only a few minutes to complete, but it can save you a lot of time when planning restorative cases and when fitting restorations.

What Does a Facebow Do?

All a facebow does is to transfer the spatial relationship of the maxillary teeth and TMJs from the patient to the articulator, enabling accurate mounting of the upper cast in relation to the joints. When the lower cast is mounted, the similarity in geometry between articulator and jaws helps to simulate the paths of jaw movement. Remember that the three main uses of articulated casts are to supplement occlusal examination, to help plan treatment through trial occlusal adjustment and diagnostic waxing and, in the laboratory, to help make restorations that will require minimal adjustment in the mouth. If you plan to undertake any of these procedures, we recommend you use a facebow.

What Are the Main Components?

Some facebows come as two main components – the bow and the bitefork – with a clamping mechanism to join the two together. This type of facebow is cumbersome to transport to the laboratory. Other facebows, such as the Denar Slidematic (Fig 8-18), have three components – the bow, the bitefork and a transfer jig. The advantage of the transfer jig is that the bow remains in the surgery for use on other patients, while the transfer jig/bitefork assembly goes to the laboratory. The DVD shows how to use this facebow clinically. The principles are the same whichever system you choose to use.

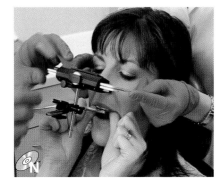

Fig 8-18 A facebow simply transfers the relationship between the maxillary teeth and the TMJs.

What Reference Points Do Facebows Use?

Facebows come in a number of designs. All of them locate to three reference points on a patient. Two of these reference points are the condyles, specifically the hinge axis running through both condyles in CR. Most modern facebows are termed "earbows", as they use the external auditory meati as stable reference points adjacent to the hinge axis. With some old designs of facebow, the bow locates over the lateral aspect of the condyles, making accurate records more difficult to obtain – the process has been likened to nailing a jellyfish to the ceiling!

The third reference point aligns the bow to the horizontal plane, with the patient sitting upright. Anatomically, this is the Frankfort plane, extending from the tragus of the ear to the infraorbital notch. Some facebows use a pointer specifically to align with the infraorbital notch. Others use different anatomical landmarks. The Whip Mix facebow uses the nasal bridge (nasion), while the third reference point for the Denar is a fixed distance, marked on the cheek with a pen, above the incisal edge of the right lateral incisor (Fig 8-19). There is no mystery to this third reference point, it ensures that the casts when mounted are centrally placed between the two members of the articulator, giving an indication of the relationship between the occlusal and the Frankfort planes.

How Accurate Are Facebows?

Facebows need to be used with care, but they do not need to be as accurate in their recording as interocclusal registrations. In practice, facebows are

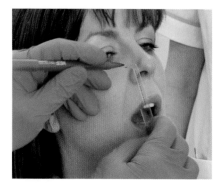

Fig 8-19 This mark, called the "third reference point", aligns the facebow to the patient's horizontal plane.

accurate to millimetres while interocclusal records need to be accurate to micrometres. Nevertheless, clinically significant inaccuracies can arise with earbow registrations for the following reasons:

- failures in recording technique
- discrepancies between the patient's hinge axis and the average values used for earbows
- facial asymmetry
- laboratory errors.

The Technique

Success with facebows is a matter of being vigilant. All the parts of the bow should be able to move freely before it is tightened. Sometimes, the clamp holding the bitefork becomes too tight because of contamination with molten wax, or an overtightened and distorted clamp makes it difficult to position the bow properly. In such cases, clean off the wax or ease the distorted clamp by loosening off the screw and levering it open. One of the most common problems is that the facebow clamps are not tightened sufficiently, so the bitefork moves before or during mounting. Finally, remember to show your nurse how to guide the earpieces into the ears properly. The bow needs to be pulled forwards as the earpieces are moved inwards. With practice the procedure becomes second nature.

Hinge Axis Discrepancies

There may be a few millimetres discrepancy between the patient's real hinge axis and that determined by an earbow. This usually does not produce any significant problems, but the rule to follow is to record the interocclusal registration at, or very close to, the vertical dimension required, thereby minimising the impact of any hinge axis discrepancy. This applies both to diagnosis and in the construction of restorations and appliances. You could use a hinge axis locator to make an extremely accurate facebow registration; however, the extra time taken to locate the patient's terminal hinge axis is of little benefit – unless you routinely use a fully adjustable articulator and fit difficult full-mouth reconstructions all at one time, but not many dentists do that.

Patients with a Facial Asymmetry

When restoring multiple anterior teeth, a facebow helps to define the occlusal plane and avoid having a "run" on the restorations. Should a patient have a significant facial asymmetry, defining the incisal level of the new restorations can be difficult. There are, however, various strategies that can be employed to take account of this.

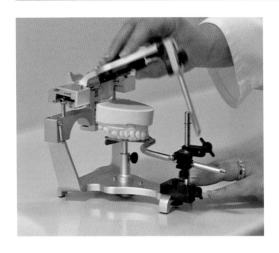

Fig 8-20 The bitefork and black transfer jig are attached to an articulator. Beneath the cast is a supporting device to prevent sagging during mounting.

Laboratory Errors

In the laboratory, the bitefork must be supported during mounting of the upper cast or it will sag. An elegant way of doing this is shown in Fig 8-20.

Do I Need to Buy a Facebow?

Some laboratories might be prepared to lend or hire a facebow for use with more advanced crown and bridgework, which is a reasonable alternative to buying one if only a limited amount of such work is undertaken. However, this approach can easily become a barrier to using a facebow. A better option is to have the equipment available in the surgery. Having an articulator in the surgery is useful for treatment planning. We consider types of articulator in the following section.

8-6 ARTICULATOR SELECTION O,P

Choosing the right articulator is critical in the planning and successful provision of restorative dentistry. The DVD details the two most useful instruments – the semi-adjustable and average value articulators (video O) – and the process of cast mounting (video P). Articulators are widely used to construct restorations, with the principal purpose of the articulator being to facilitate the construction of restorations that will require little, if any, chair-side occlusal adjustment. In contrast, articulators are not widely used for diagnostic purposes.

An articulator is simply a device to which casts are attached to allow simulation of jaw position and movement. Without a facebow registration, the best articulator in the world would be unable to simulate the paths of movement of the jaw or reproduce the angulation of the occlusal plane. It is at the tooth level that jaw movement assumes major importance. A significant difference in jaw movement between patient and articulator will cause misdiagnoses or lead to restorations blighted by deflective contacts and interferences.

Articulators are easily classified according to how well they simulate jaw movement, which in turn is influenced by their complexity and the degree of skill needed to operate them. Articulators can be classified as follows:
• simple hinge
• small crown and bridge
• average value
• semi-adjustable
• fully adjustable
• fossa moulding.

A summary of advice on articulator selection for different clinical applications is given in Table 8-2.

The main components of articulators comprise the upper and lower members, which simulate the upper and lower jaws. Attached to the members are the condylar and fossa elements. Most articulators use plaster (preferably with anti-expansion solution) for mounting casts, but a few designs do not. A plasterless articulator popular in some laboratories is the Galetti. Although convenient to use, this type of articulator is not without problems, both in terms of holding casts dependably and simulating jaw movement (Fig 8-21).

Table 8-2 **Advice on articulator selection and appropriate occlusal records**

Situation	Articulator choice	Records
Diagnosis		
Occlusal analysis *Trial occlusal adjustment* *Diagnostic waxing*	Average value or semi-adjustable	Facebow, CR or ICP record as appropriate
Restorations		
Single posterior restoration	Hand-held casts, small crown and bridge	ICP record
Multiple posterior restorations (with posterior disclusion)	Average value	Facebow, ICP record
Multiple posterior restorations (with group function)	Semi-adjustable	Facebow, ICP record, optional lateral check record (if group function being waxed for whole sextant)
Single upper anterior restoration	Hand-held casts (if guidance can be developed from adjacent teeth) or average value	ICP record, pretreatment casts if guidance cannot be developed from adjacent teeth
Multiple upper anterior restorations	Average value or semi-adjustable	Facebow, ICP record, pretreatment casts (from which to copy guidance), impression of provisional restorations resulting from diagnostic wax-up
Full arch	Average value or semi-adjustable (if canine guidance achievable) Fully adjustable if shallow guidance from posterior teeth and bruxism	As for multiple and anterior restorations CR record at correct occlusal vertical dimension plus mechanical or electronic pantographic record

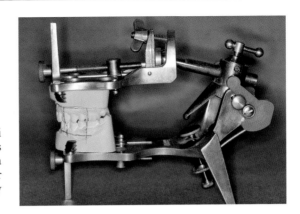

Fig 8-21 The Galetti plasterless articulator. This cannot be used with a facebow as its condylar elements are geometrically in the wrong place.

What Is Most Important in Articulator Accuracy?

Whichever type of articulator is used, the most important considerations are always an accurate set of casts and accurate mounting in either ICP or CR. The best articulator cannot compensate for poor casts or inaccurate mounting.

Simple articulators, such as the hinge articulator (Fig 8-22) or small crown and bridge articulator, are adequate to relate casts in ICP, but they provide either no or limited simulation of jaw movement. In addition, they are unable to accept a facebow transfer and, therefore, are useless for CR mountings. At the other end of the spectrum, the fully adjustable and fossa moulding articulators give superb replication of mandibular border movements, but

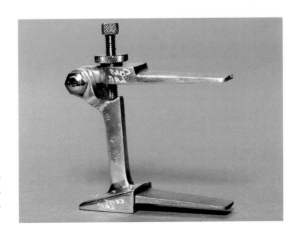

Fig 8-22 A simple hinge articulator, which has limited application in restorative dentistry.

these take considerable time and skill to programme, usually for little additional gain. For most restorative purposes, semi-adjustable articulators represent the optimum choice, giving an adequate simulation of mandibular movement for most patients without being excessively complex. Given that semi-adjustable articulators are often used with the settings adjusted to an average value, many cases can be mounted on a less-expensive average value articulator which has the capacity to accept a facebow transfer. The following sections consider semi-adjustable and average value articulators.

Semi-adjustable and Average Value Articulators

The DVD (video O) shows the dynamics of these two types of articulator. Articulators are broadly classified as arcon and non-arcon. "Arcon" is an abbreviation of "articulating condyle", which means the articulator has its condylar elements attached to its lower member, as occurs naturally. As such, the articulator elements in an arcon articulator resemble simplified TMJs (Fig 8-23). With non-arcon instruments, the condylar elements are attached to the upper member (Fig 8-24).

Arcon articulators (e.g. Denar Mk II, Whip Mix, Kavo Protar) are preferred for occlusal analysis and crown and bridgework as the upper member can be easily detached, facilitating such work. Non-arcon articulators (e.g. Dentatus, Hanau) are preferred for denture construction as the upper and lower members in most models remain hinged together. This is an advantage in the laboratory.

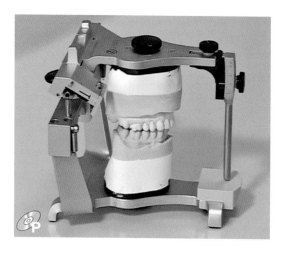

Fig 8-23 The Denar Mk II, a workhorse of restorative dentistry, is a semi-adjustable arcon articulator. The condylar elements are attached to the lower member, as in life.

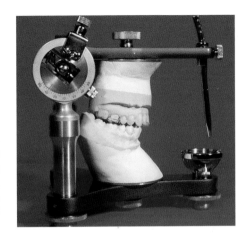

Fig 8-24 The Dentatus, a non-arcon articulator often preferred for denture work. The fossa elements are attached to the lower member, making it difficult, if not impossible, to separate the upper and lower members.

Non-arcon semi-adjustable articulators rely on three surfaces within each fossa element to guide excursive movements – the superior, medial and rear walls. Not all semi-adjustable articulators have the same adjustments. Generally, all have adjustments for the height of the incisal guide pin and condylar guidance angle. Depending on the model, there may also be adjustments for progressive and immediate side shifts, which dictate the character of lateral excursive movements.

If you have not already done so, you should watch the DVD, which clearly shows how the condyles move in lateral excursions. Once you have seen the condyles move in lateral excursion, the concept of progressive side shift is easy to understand. For the sake of completeness, *progressive side shift is sideways movement of the mandible occurring at a rate proportional to the forwards movement of the orbiting condyle.* This occurs as the orbiting condylar element slides against the medial wall of the fossa element and the rotating condylar element slides outwards along the posterior wall. The angulation of the medial wall to the sagittal plane determines the amount of progressive side shift. Progressive side shift is often confused as being synonymous with the Bennett angle. In fact, the Bennett angle measures the combination of progressive and immediate side shift. In practical terms, these aspects of occlusion are relatively unimportant.

Immediate side shift, confusingly also called "Bennett movement", is essentially a small amount of "slop" in the fit of the condyles within their fossae, such that the whole mandible moves sideways immediately on lateral excursion. It occurs only in some, generally older patients, suggesting it represents a degree of wear and tear. If it happens, it occurs during the first 4 mm of lateral excursion, amounting to around 0.5–1.5 mm of movement. As the direction and timing of the movement are difficult to simulate accurately, the value of including an immediate side shift adjustment on an articulator has been questioned, unless a mechanical or electronic pantograph (e.g. Denar Cadiax, Kavo Arcus Digma) is used to programme the instrument. If no account is taken of immediate side shift, the paths of movement at tooth level, especially across the posterior teeth, may differ slightly between patient and articulator. This is not of critical importance and is of little consequence if the anterior teeth provide guidance and posteriorly there are relatively shallow cusps that disclude during excursions.

Another adjustment seen on fully adjustable articulators which is of limited value to semi-adjustable articulators (some of which include it) is intercondylar distance. Constantly moving the condylar elements between settings causes the components to wear, resulting in loss of overall mounting accuracy. For this reason, most modern articulators simply have a medium intercondylar width of 110 mm and accept a small sacrifice in the accuracy of the simulated lateral excursions.

Finally, a further difference between arcon articulators is whether straight or curved surfaces are used for the guiding surfaces of the fossa elements. In life, patients' condyles follow curves rather than straight lines, but these curves vary considerably between patients.

In most situations, the limitations of not having a perfect anatomical representation – because of the lack of a curved condylar path, an exact match for intercondylar distance or a precise simulation of immediate side shift – make little real difference to appropriate diagnosis and the construction of restorations. Average value and semi-adjustable articulators provide sufficient representation of functional movements when used properly.

How Do I Set a Semi-adjustable Articulator?

Many textbooks advise the use of "check bites" for setting condylar angles in semi-adjustable articulators. Check bites are wax or silicone occlusal records recorded in lateral and protrusive excursions. These records are transferred to the articulator and used to adjust the superior and medial walls of the fossa elements. The idea is to maintain contact with the condylar balls during excursions. In reality, this technique is highly error prone, although it may be a reasonable approach for constructing restorations in group function.

Many experienced operators prefer to use "average value" settings for most situations. Typically, these would be 25° condylar guidance and 7° progressive side shift. A condylar guidance angle of 25° is lower than averages measured in real life, bearing in mind the limitations of measuring angles along curved paths, but it is chosen for good reason. Restorations should be made with relatively shallow cusps and when fitted must not clash during excursions. Denar has incorporated these angles in the fossae of its average value articulator.

Facets on unrestored teeth can give a clue as to the paths of mandibular movement at tooth level. It is often possible to adjust semi-adjustable articulators to allow these facets to contact in excursions. Clearly, such provision is not available in an average value instrument.

Is a Fully Adjustable Articulator Ever Needed?

The short answer for most dentists is no. Fully adjustable articulators and jaw-tracking instruments seduce many who have attended courses or have read about such technology. Once the initial enthusiasm has waned, much of this expensive kit becomes redundant. In fact, almost all cases can be managed with a semi-adjustable articulator. However, to avoid the possibility of multiple adjustments of restorations, each case should be broken down to limit the number of restorations fitted at each stage. This approach is described in Chapter 4.

One situation where using average values could give rise to problems is in the full-mouth rehabilitation of bruxists with limited anterior guidance, as a consequence of a Class III incisal relationship (Fig 8-25). Here, the potential for posterior disclusion is limited or non-existent. Therefore, the posterior teeth often have to provide guidance, and being closer to the TMJs than the anterior teeth there is a need to have an accurate simulation of condylar movement, particularly if immediate side shift is present. This is possible with a fully adjustable articulator because each fossa element can be tailored to the individual patient using a pantographic record (Fig 8-26).

A summary of advice on articulator selection for different clinical applications is given in Table 8-2.

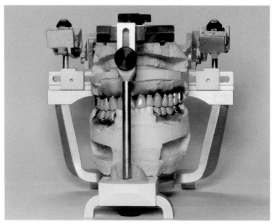

Fig 8-25 A Denar fully adjustable articulator set up using a pantograph, being used in a case of full-mouth reconstruction for a bruxist with a Class III incisor relationship.

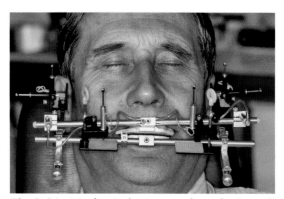

Fig 8-26 Mechanical pantograph with six styli attached to an upper facebow. The styli scribe mandibular movement onto six tables attached to the lower facebow. The assembly is transferred to the fully adjustable articulator, which is adjusted to follow the scribed paths. Electronic pantographs provide a list of settings, which simplifies the process of articulator programming.

8-7 Occlusal Adjustment/Equilibration Q-S

The DVD gives the clinical context to this often misunderstood technique. It is suggested that you view the relevant tracks before reading this section.

The DVD shows a patient with functional occlusal problems who was treated by occlusal equilibration. The three video tracks relevant to this section are:
- Q – Occlusal analysis (on mounted casts)
- R – Trial occlusal adjustment (on mounted casts)
- S – Clinical occlusal adjustment and follow-up.

Why Are Dentists Cautious about Adjusting Occlusions?

Many dentists are fearful about undertaking occlusal adjustments for their patients. This probably stems from a combination of a lack of practical teaching, a fear of causing problems and the knowledge that occlusal adjustment is not supported scientifically as a mainstay of treatment, in particular in the management of TMDs.

While most patients adapt to occlusal changes and discrepancies, some do have problems associated with deflective contacts and interferences and may benefit from adjustment. Furthermore, when restoring patients with, for example, deflective contacts, it is necessary to decide whether to conform and accept them, or to reorganise the occlusion to eliminate them. Unfortunately, it is difficult to design randomised controlled trials to help when making these decisions.

A word of caution before looking at the practicalities of occlusal adjustment: unless you have a good restorative reason, or there is a problem that appears to be clearly linked to the occlusion, think twice before committing yourself (Table 8-3). Fortunately, in many cases the treatment is neither difficult nor risky, and a balance between caution and confidence is reasonable.

Adjustment and Equilibration – What is the Difference?

Occlusal adjustment and equilibration are defined as follows:
- *Occlusal adjustment* is any alteration of the occluding surfaces of the teeth or restorations.
- *Occlusal equilibration* is the modification of the occlusal forms of the teeth, with the intent of equalising occlusal stress, producing simultaneous contacts or harmonising cuspal relations.

119

Table 8-3 **Features of patients sensitive to occlusal changes**

The "Picky Patient"
Some patients will adapt to just about any occlusal change, but others are highly sensitive to a discrepancy of just a few micrometres. Careful occlusal examination usually shows these discerning patients to be correct in their perception. Adjustments are necessarily time consuming but are usually successful

"Phantom Bite"
This unusual problem normally starts after dental work involving occlusal surfaces. Patients have the following characteristics: • utterly preoccupied with the way their teeth meet • symptoms described in an often exaggerated and bizarre way, sometimes with written and drawn explanations • symptoms may not match with the dentist's examination findings.   Subsequent occlusal adjustments are ineffective and may worsen the condition, with the patient moving from dentist to dentist in search of a physical cure. It is a poorly understood disorder of perception and notoriously difficult to treat effectively. Patients are best referred for specialist dental and, where available and where acceptable to the patient, psychological management

Occlusal adjustment and equilibration are usually considered subtractive processes, in that they involve grinding away tooth or restoration. It is also possible to modify the occlusion by additive means through the provision of occlusal restoration or a reconstruction.

Occlusal equilibration is in essence a type of occlusal adjustment. It can be simple, complex or anything in between. This will depend on the size and nature of the discrepancy between RCP and ICP, the amount of excursive interference and the number of teeth needing adjustment. Teeth are usually equilibrated around CR. In a healthy masticatory system, CR is relatively stable, provides comfortable function and can be reliably transferred to an articulator – which is why we use it. With dysfunctional TMJs and muscles, CR is often unstable. The dysfunction must be treated before even considering an occlusal equilibration.

As with occlusal equilibration, occlusal adjustments can be simple, complex or anything in between. A simple adjustment might involve the elimination of a small deflective contact or interference on a single tooth, or a small number of teeth, with minimal change in jaw relationship. A complex adjustment might involve part or all of a more demanding equilibration: for instance, the elimination of deflective contacts significantly affecting mandibular alignment between CR and ICP. Clinically, it may be sufficient to stop the adjustment once you have eliminated the slide. Alternatively, you may decide to go on to refine the new occlusal scheme by removing excursive interferences and refining guidance. In some cases, this may be more than is required, but provided the adjustment is not unnecessarily destructive, it is reassuring to know that you have eliminated potentially damaging influences – what might be termed "occlusal hygiene"!

What Are the Indications for Simple Occlusal Adjustment?

Simple adjustment may be appropriate to reduce heavy occlusal loading that has resulted in tooth pain, fracture (Figs 8-27 and 8-28), a cracked cusp or mobility (Chapter 5). A simple occlusal adjustment may also be a good way to create interocclusal space for a restoration, notably when overeruption has produced minor discrepancies in the occlusal plane. At all times keep in mind the potential to expose sensitive dentine, which may limit the amount of adjustment possible or necessitate additional restoration.

In Chapter 3, the effects of pivoting contacts were considered. If these pivots are inadvertently removed during crown preparation, a loss of interocclusal space can result. One way of managing this problem is to adjust the pivot prior to preparation. In some situations this is relatively simple, involving only a single pair of teeth, but in others a more complex adjustment may be required. Therefore, should you need to crown a tooth involved in a pivoting contact, it is best first to mount diagnostic casts and carry out a trial adjustment before committing to a possibly difficult procedure.

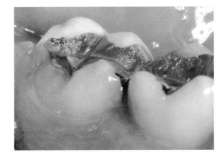

Fig 8-27 Fracture of lingual cusps occurs commonly in restored molars. Often these cusps stand proud without any holding contact. Simply shortening them or onlaying the restoration may reduce their vulnerability to damage.

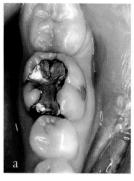
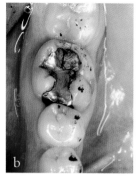

Fig 8-28a
Fractured amalgam in first molar showing signs of occlusal overload.

Fig 8-28b
Mark with articulating foil to show excursive contacts (*red*) and holding contacts (*black*).

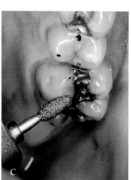
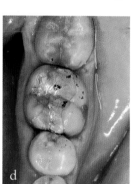

Fig 8-28c
Shorten overerupted opposing cusp to eliminate non-working interference.

Fig 8-28d
Build amalgam back into contact, but without damaging interferences.

What Are the Indications for More Complex Adjustment?

The adjustment becomes more complex when multiple teeth are involved, or in situations in which the jaw relationship is changed to give a new, hopefully more stable, ICP. Listed below are situations where you might consider equilibrating the teeth to eliminate deflective contacts and interferences:

- **To relieve dental pain** (Fig 8-29): Here you need to be confident of an accurate diagnosis of heavy occlusal loading – teeth showing fremitus, heavy occlusal contact markings and shim stock contacts that are obviously firmer than on adjacent teeth. Remember that patients with unexplained dental pain may have neuropathic pain or atypical odontalgia, which would not be expected to respond to occlusal adjustment over the longer term. Therefore, do not start an adjustment unless your clinical findings confirm adverse occlusal contacts which the patient would benefit from having removed.

Fig 8-29 More than a year after fitting this crown, the patient still suffered pain and a feeling that the "bite was not right".

Adjustment necessitated grinding through to metal and resulted in the heavy contact moving to the second premolar. The high crown had resulted in occlusal instability through minor movement of several teeth.

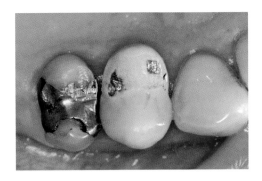

- **To eliminate an anterior thrust** (Fig 8-30a,b): This thrust may cause localised discomfort, wear, drifting, mobility or fractured/decemented restorations. The equilibration shown on the DVD is for an anterior thrust arising from occlusal instability. Often, an anterior thrust results from the mandible being forced forwards or laterally during closure by a single deflective contact, but you may need to adjust many teeth to eliminate the RCP–ICP slide.

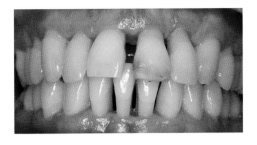

Fig 8-30a Drifting of maxillary incisors is often associated with periodontal disease, but this patient also had an anterior thrust caused by posterior deflective contacts.

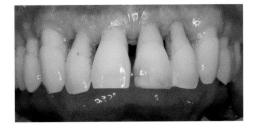

Fig 8-30b Following periodontal treatment, equilibration resulted in a reduction of incisor fremitus and partial closure of the diastema.

- **To provide space for anterior restorations:** "Distalisation of the mandible" is only possible if there is a relatively large horizontal component in the RCP–ICP slide, with the mandible translating bodily between the two positions. On elimination of the slide, space is created between the upper and lower anterior teeth. This is discussed in Section 8-11.

- **To provide posterior stability as part of a reorganised occlusal reconstruction:** For example to:
  - facilitate jaw manipulation and registration
  - prevent mandibular repositioning during preparation or temporisation following removal of pivoting contacts
  - avoid inadvertently incorporating deflective contacts in the new restorations.

- **In the management of TMD:** As discussed in Chapter 7, extensive adjustment or full equilibration may occasionally be justified after splint therapy.

- **For management of bruxism** (Fig 8-31a–d): As discussed in Chapter 3, nocturnal bruxism is a sleep-related disorder and there is little evidence to support occlusal adjustment as being effective management. Nevertheless, patients who are aware of tooth grinding on an uncomfortable contact may benefit from occlusal adjustment or equilibration. Although not providing a cure for bruxism, there may be merit in adjusting or equilibrating to improve the occlusal load distribution during excursions. For instance, a patient who has a post crown on a canine may have canine guidance converted to a group function to protect the canine from damage. Such adjustments need to be planned and executed very carefully to ensure one set of occlusal discrepancies is not substituted for another.

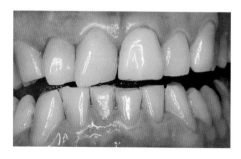

Fig 8-31a A patient with a daytime bruxing habit against the elongated distal aspect of the upper right incisor.

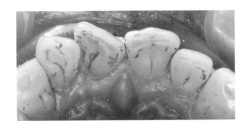

Fig 8-31b There was a heavy contact mesially on this tooth.

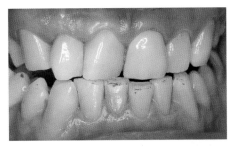

Fig 8-31c The incisor was adjusted to spread the load more evenly across the incisal edges.

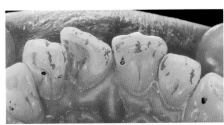

Fig 8-31d The incisor adjusted to spread the load across the lingual aspects.

What Are the Aims of Occlusal Adjustment/Equilibration?

There are two main aims in carrying out an occlusal adjustment or equilibration:
• To improve the distribution of occlusal forces through the restorations, teeth, periodontium and TMJs.
• To provide an occlusal scheme within a patient's neuromuscular adaptive capacity.

How Do I Achieve These Aims?
Choose a jaw relationship
The first thing to decide is whether you are going to maintain the existing intercuspal jaw relationship or use CR as your starting point. In the case of a minor occlusal adjustment, you should generally conform to the existing ICP.

If the intention is to eliminate a deflective contact on the hinge axis, then the primary aim of the adjustment will be to produce a new, stable ICP that is coincident with CR – in other words, to reorganise. If there is any doubt over the stability of CR, or if the patient has signs of TMD, a stabilisation splint should be provided before equilibration and adjusted over a period of time until a stable set of contacts is obtained. Alternatively, if the patient requires extensive crown work, you may prescribe a period of prolonged temporisation, again adjusting until the occlusion is stable.

Decide on the intercuspal contacts
Should you decide to equilibrate, you need to have a clear idea of the new ICP contacts. ICP should occur in CR. The contacts should be multiple, simultaneous, small and positioned to direct occlusal forces down the long axes of the teeth to prevent unwanted tooth movement. This can be difficult to achieve, but the thing to avoid on posterior teeth is having a single contact on a sloping cuspal incline. In such situations, the teeth can overerupt and eventually slip into an interfering relationship.

It is reasonable to regard the adjustment as complete once a stable ICP is achieved which is coincident with CR. If you want to progress to a full equilibration, the excursive contacts need to be addressed.

Adjust excursive contacts
These should be to a predetermined scheme. Ideally, the contacts should be smooth and not interfere with mandibular movement, be between teeth capable of sustaining them, and involve compatible materials, avoiding those that may wear (unpolished porcelain) or be easily worn (glass ionomer).

Preferably, lateral excursive contacts should be on the working side only. Classically, the excursive contacts are either canine guided or group function, but in some cases it is impossible to achieve either of these schemes by simply grinding the teeth. A smooth, harmonious contact between a pair of working-side premolars, or even molars, is often acceptable. Where such guidance is unacceptable, restorations such as canine ramps of metal or composite can provide satisfactory guidance.

Non-working-side contacts are not necessary for function. They are usually innocuous and do not need to be removed. Nevertheless, they can be eliminated if you suspect they are causing problems or where you want to avoid reintroducing them into restorations.

Aim for mutually protected occlusion

This occurs frequently in natural dentitions and is an aspiration following equilibrium. In ICP, the posterior teeth support axially directed forces while the anterior teeth are in light contact. The anterior teeth, which are best suited to accept nonaxial forces, provide guidance while the posterior teeth are discluded. When occlusal adjustment or equilibrium is being considered it is often possible, and indeed desirable, to provide such an occlusal scheme. To see a mutually protected occlusion, look again at animations A, B and C on the DVD.

Planning Occlusal Adjustments/Equilibration

Minor occlusal adjustments can be undertaken after careful examination, but more extensive adjustments, let alone full equilibrations, need a more considered approach. This entails a clinical occlusal examination together with an examination of study casts mounted on an articulator by means of a facebow and a CR jaw record. Two sets of casts allow one set to be used to practise adjustments, as shown on the DVD, while the other can be kept as a medicolegal record. The pattern of adjustment can best be mapped out if the occlusal surfaces of the teeth are first painted with a thin coat of paint or thinned die spacer (Fig 8-32). Thin articulating foil (e.g. GHM Occlusion Prüf Folie, Germany) and shim stock should be used to mark the occlusal contacts and a sharp blade or bur used to make the trial adjustment.

When practising an equilibration on study casts, you should try to answer three simple questions:
- Is it possible?
- Is it stable?
- Is it sensible?

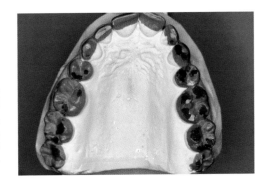

Fig 8-32 Paint the occlusal surfaces to show the location and amount of adjustment: (*blue*, deflective contact removal; *yellow*, adjusted excursive contacts). This is an excellent way to assist learning.

Clearly, if the adjustment is not going to be a practical solution, it is best to find this out on the casts. Other options for providing occlusal stability may then be considered, including occlusal restorations, orthodontics, surgery or prolonged stabilisation splint wear.

Some adjustments are much easier to carry out than others. For instance, where the patient has an RCP–ICP slide with a large vertical and small horizontal component, the equilibration may only involve one tooth and be carried out simply. By contrast, a slide with a large horizontal or, in particular, a lateral component may involve several teeth, and, depending on the amount of mandibular translation, substantial tooth reduction may be required. This is not the type of case you want to start on!

A useful way of assessing the amount of mandibular translation between RCP and ICP is to view the gap that results between the articulator's condylar elements and the posterior wall of the fossa elements, as shown on the DVD. Where there are horizontal or lateral components of slide, the equilibration should produce a small flat area of contact between RCP and ICP – long and wide centric respectively.

To avoid an ineffective and destructive adjustment, it is extremely important to know:

- the directions teeth move across each other during excursions – look at the "crow's foot" animation associated with Chapter 2 (DVD track D)
- the cuspal inclines involved with deflective contacts and interferences (Table 8-4).

Procedure on Casts

Providing a Stable ICP
Remove any deflective contacts and establish a new ICP which is stable and coincident with CR. Sometimes, after removing deflective contacts with a horizontal component of slide, the mandible repositions posteriorly. As it does, the cusp/fossa relationships become less than ideal, with the adjusted contacts peripherally sited on the posterior teeth. Therefore it may be necessary to "warp" the shapes of the upper and lower cusps to bring the contacts more centrally into the fossae. It may be appropriate to stop the adjustment at this point.

Progressing to Excursive Movements
After the deflective contacts have been eliminated, a decision needs to be made about whether to progress to full equilibration, specifically the removal

Table 8-4 **Cuspal inclines involved with deflective contacts and interferences**

Problem	Maxillary cusp incline	Mandibular cusp incline
Deflective contact[1]	Mesial facing	Distal facing
Non-working-side interference	Buccal facing	Lingual facing
Working-side interference	Lingual facing	Buccal facing
Protrusive interference	Distal facing	Mesial facing

Notes:
1. Deflective contacts, which produce a lateral component of slide, will also involve the buccal- or lingual-facing inclines of the upper and lower teeth.

of working, non-working and protrusive interferences. This takes time and skill and the decision will depend on whether you feel there is any advantage to doing so; for example, evidence of damage to teeth or symptoms that may justify this. It may also depend on what you find when you adjust the casts. What follows is really the small print of occlusal adjustment, but is important if you want to progress to this stage.

The first decision is whether the anterior guidance is to be immediate or delayed. An immediate anterior guidance provides instant disclusion of the posterior teeth. In a delayed guidance, the posterior teeth move across small flat areas of adjusted occlusal contact before disclusion takes place. A rule of thumb is that the small flat areas should be less than 1 mm in length anteroposteriorly or mediolaterally. As these small flat areas are difficult to refine, it is generally easier to equilibrate the occlusion, if immediate guidance can be provided. If not, the following options are available:

- Adjust posterior teeth to close the vertical dimension slightly, thus bringing canines/incisors into contact to provide immediate guidance.
- Accept delayed guidance and use premolars instead of canines to guide lateral excursions.
- Restore lingual surfaces of upper canines/incisors with guidance ramps using either shims or crowns.

What Do I Tell the Patient?

Patients need to be able to appreciate what you are trying to achieve by the proposed occlusal adjustment. It does, after all, involve the rather disconcerting grinding away of precious and irreplaceable tooth tissue. They need to know and accept the inherent risks. These will be different in every case and in some cases may not be significant. The risks include:

- dentine sensitivity, usually transient but may need further treatment
- crown perforation or disruption of plastic restorations, which may need replacement
- awareness of changed occlusal contact (though this is often a positive change for the patient)
- jaw soreness or headache as the neuromuscular system accommodates
- slight roughness of tooth contact, which will usually self-polish with time unless no attempt has been made to smooth adjusted enamel with fine diamond or tungsten carbide burs.

Furthermore, patients need to appreciate that one or more follow-up appointments, depending on complexity, might be necessary to refine the adjustment.

Often, patients attend the adjustment appointment with further questions about the procedure. The vast majority of patients will accept a recommendation for an adjustment, provided it is carefully explained (Fig 8-33).

On no account should an occlusal adjustment/equilibration be undertaken without the patient's informed consent.

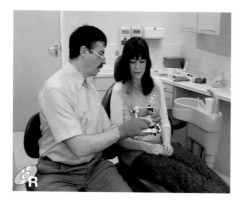

Fig 8-33 Being able to show patients the trial adjustment is indispensable to securing informed consent.

8-8 DIAGNOSTIC WAXING AND RELATED TECHNIQUES

The aim of this section is to explain how wax-ups are produced and to consider their many diagnostic and therapeutic uses. Diagnostic tools such as the wax-up are particularly indispensable when planning complex cases. They allow an end point to be visualised at the outset which forms the basis of communication with technician and patient. This section can be read in conjunction with Chapter 4 on conformative and reorganised occlusal schemes.

A wax-up is where changes are made to the shapes of teeth by adding wax to stone models of the patient's dental arch. The purpose of the wax-up may simply be to visualise the effects of aesthetic restorations, such as using composite resin to close a diastema. However, wax-ups can be used for a great deal more than this, particularly when mounted on a semi-adjustable articulator. This allows the simulation of different occlusal schemes and the assessment of the need for restorations. As part of wider treatment planning, wax-ups are invaluable when the occlusion is to be reorganised.

It is important to appreciate that creating wax-ups is not just about adding wax – subtractive adjustments, including the removal of deflective contacts and shortening of overerupted teeth, can also be simulated. Creating a wax-up is an evolutionary process, with treatment options becoming evident as the work progresses. Strictly speaking, only the clinician is in a position to decide how much adjustment or addition to existing teeth can be realistically simulated. However, good communication with a technician who understands the constraints can be effective, and has the advantage of engaging the technician from the outset of the case.

Uses of Diagnostic Wax-ups

On theoretical grounds, it is hard to argue against the need for a wax-up every time the form of a tooth is to be changed, let alone when a tooth is to be replaced by bridgework or an implant. In practical terms, wax-ups are mostly used when the changes planned are likely to have a substantial impact on occlusion, aesthetics, phonetics, or hygiene. It is not the purpose of this book to consider aesthetic or phonetic aspects in any detail. Suffice it to say, occlusal, aesthetic and phonetic considerations are intimately related during all stages of dental management – change some feature of one and you may well affect another.

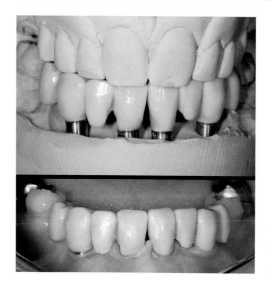

Fig 8-34 A wax-up, produced directly on implant components, has been screwed into place to verify both occlusal and aesthetic features as well as the accuracy of the cast for this patient with congenitally missing teeth.

Communication

A well-executed wax-up serves as a useful tool for communicating a treatment option to both the patient and the technician. Quite how helpful wax-ups are for patients will vary from case to case and from patient to patient. Remember, patients are not used to seeing their teeth other than when reflected in a mirror! For the patient shown in Fig 8-34, it was possible to place the wax-up in the mouth, akin to a try-in of a denture – a luxury only really possible for implant-retained restorations.

Diagnostic

The potential use of diagnostic wax-ups for aesthetic analysis is evident but beyond the scope of this book. The main considerations here are the many static and dynamic occlusal features that can be examined using wax-ups, including the following:

- scope for being able to provide stable posterior interocclusal contacts can be determined (Fig 8-35)
- adequacy of crown height for effective resistance and retention, or the need to create interocclusal space by some means
- interincisal relationship and any need to accentuate the cingulum area of maxillary teeth to achieve contact (Fig 8-36), particularly when planning an increase in occlusal vertical dimension
- scope for being able to create or maintain the prosthodontic advantages of canine guidance (Fig 8-37)

- ability to avoid non-working-side interferences in proposed restorations
- steepness of dynamic contacts between anterior teeth – anterior tooth guidance.

Fig 8-35 This wax-up has been made in preparation for providing cusp-covering indirect restorations for heavily restored posterior dentition (which includes various deteriorating plastic restorations).

Among other things, the wax-up shows that stable occlusal contacts are achievable.

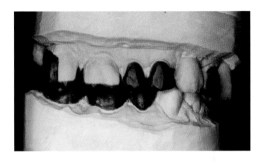

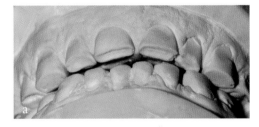

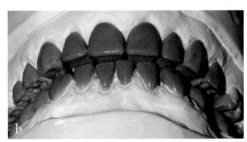

Fig 8-36 (a–c) A wax-up has been carried out to investigate the possibility of capturing inter-incisal contact and guidance for this patient with tooth wear.

The wax-up has been carried out at an increased vertical dimension of occlusion. This has accentuated the overjet, resulting in the pronounced cingulum contours to maintain occlusal stability.

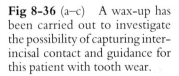

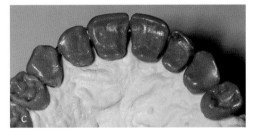

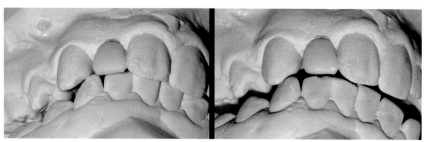

Fig 8-37 This simple wax-up shows that it is possible to avoid right lateral excursive contact on the maxillary lateral incisor. This may be desirable if the tooth is to be replaced with an implant.

Moving On to Treatment

Once a diagnostic wax-up has been used to establish a plan, the information contained in it can facilitate the subsequent treatment. This may be limited to the laboratory using the wax-up to create the desired outcome, or the wax-up may be used to produce matrices for the following purposes:

- to guide tooth preparation (Fig 8-38) or the construction of a custom implant abutment
- for the production of provisional restorations, both at the chair-side and in the laboratory (Fig 8-39)
- to form composite restorations – a silicone putty matrix is especially useful for establishing the palatal contour of anterior teeth (Fig 8-40)
- to assess the position of implants in relation to planned tooth positions
- to guide the technician in producing the final restorations, according to the predetermined form.

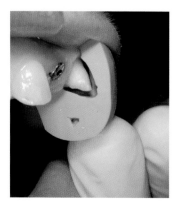

Fig 8-38 A silicone putty matrix formed over a diagnostic wax-up is being used to guide aesthetic and occlusal reduction for a full-coverage crown.

- to provide the outline form for the production of radiopaque scan appliances for implant planning and implant surgical guides (Fig 8-41).

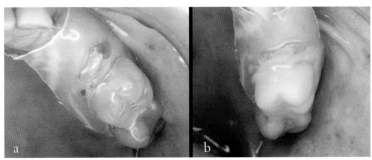

Fig 8-39 (a) A vacuum-formed shell has been made over a cast of a diagnostic wax-up for a maxillary molar. (b) The shell filled with provisional crown and bridge material to make a provisional full-coverage crown.

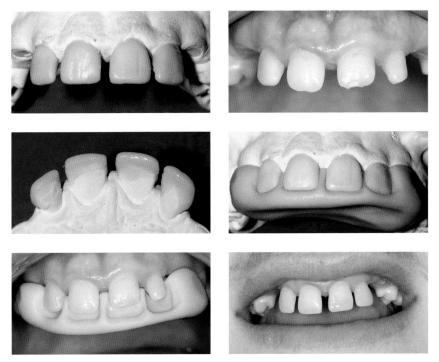

Fig 8-40 A silicone putty matrix formed over a diagnostic wax-up is used to guide composite additions to microdont teeth, both for aesthetic and occlusal contours.

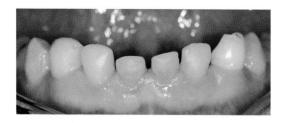

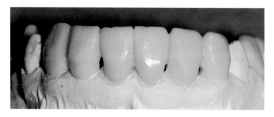

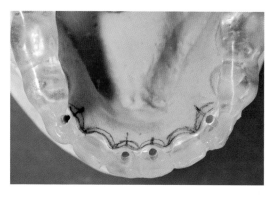

Fig 8-41 A diagnostic wax-up has been used to make a guide for implant placement. The patient has retained deciduous teeth in the anterior mandible with no permanent successors.

Requirements, Materials and Techniques for Producing Wax-ups

As with any laboratory work, high-quality casts are required. The casts should be meticulously prepared and as free from voids and bubbles as possible.

If a full occlusal analysis is to be undertaken prior to the wax-up, a CR jaw registration and facebow record will be needed. If a conformative approach has already been decided on, then it must be possible to articulate the casts accurately in ICP (Section 8-3).

Because stone casts are prone to abrasion, application of stone hardener will help to maintain tooth form during repeated excursions. It is helpful and prudent to retain a set of unmodified casts.

There are differing opinions about whether wax-ups are best made from tooth-coloured or vivid-coloured wax. The argument for vivid-coloured wax is that it helps to assess contours and visualise occlusal contacts when using marking dust. The counter-argument is that patients are more likely to relate to a tooth-coloured appearance.

Wax-ups can be produced using either a carving back technique or a wax additive technique. PK Thomas popularised an additive technique, which advocates building up the anatomy in a systematic way to form the functional features of the tooth or teeth. This technique is especially suited to posterior teeth, and if done "by the book" avoids any carving back whatsoever (Fig 8-42). It is possible to create wax-ups with stable tripod interocclusal contacts using the additive technique. This is almost impossible using the carve back technique. In reality, many technicians skilfully combine additive and carve back techniques to optimise form with precision and speed.

Sisters of the Wax-up

Trial Dentures
In addition to wax-ups, it is sometimes possible to examine features of potential occlusal schemes using a wax trial or definitive denture (Fig 8-43). This approach also gives very useful information about aesthetic options.

Intraoral Wax Trial
It may be possible to try a wax-up directly in the mouth. This is only really possible if placed over full-coverage tooth or implant preparations (Fig 8-34, page 132). This technique is unlikely to be used as the starting point of a plan, but rather to check a detail.

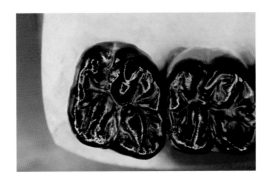

Fig 8-42 Two molars waxed up using the PK Thomas additive technique.

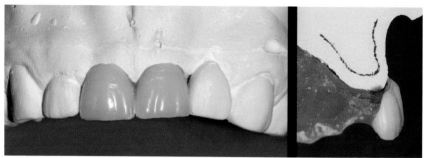

Fig 8-43 This trial denture produced satisfactory anterior occlusion and has been used further to plan the positioning of implants. The placement of the implants can proceed in the full knowledge that the external contours of the prosthetic teeth will fit the proposed occlusal scheme.

Orthodontic Planning Models (Kesling Set-ups)

It can be helpful when planning orthodontic tooth movements to modify stone casts to show final tooth position. Occlusal analysis of final tooth position is also possible by this means (Fig 8-44).

Orthodontic planning models can be further modified by wax-up and trial adjustment on the stone teeth if necessary.

Intraoral Composite Trial

This technique allows temporary additive modifications to be made directly to teeth. In its simplest form, non-bonded composite can be sculpted freehand onto teeth, allowing occlusal and aesthetic options to be evaluated. A refinement of the technique utilises a matrix made on a diagnostic wax-up to form temporary composite-resin modifications.

Alternatively, a laboratory-made acrylic mock-up can be used. This approach is sometimes helpful in deciding the length and shape of porcelain veneers.

Virtual Implant Placement

Conventional computer tomography, or cone beam volumetric tomography, allows detailed sectional and three-dimensional images of the jaws to be obtained. The usefulness of the images is greatly enhanced if a "scan appliance" is worn during the imaging; radiopaque teeth are placed in the appliance in

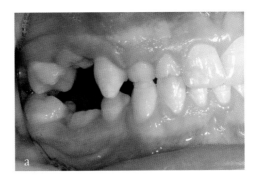

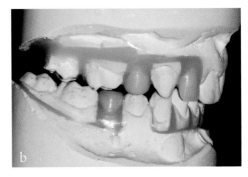

Fig 8-44 (a–c) Orthodontic planning models have been produced for this patient with multiple congenitally missing teeth. The analysis has been used to examine the potential for both maintaining canine guidance and avoiding excursive contacts on possible implant-borne tooth replacements. Part (c) shows the right working-side excursion.

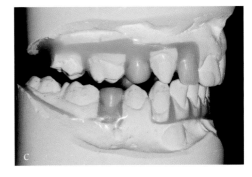

the proposed arrangement. Several software applications are available that enable virtual implant placement to be carried out on the tomographic images. Occlusal possibilities can be analysed by adding virtual abutments to the implants and by careful reference to the contours of the radiopaque teeth (Fig 8-45).

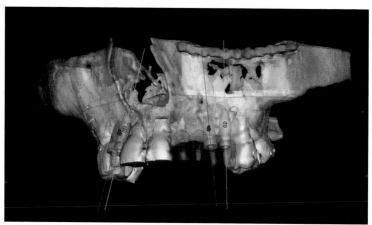

Fig 8-45 Virtual implants and abutments have been placed in this three-dimensional image so that they emerge within the confines of the radiopaque scan appliance (coloured pink). As long as the contours of the scan appliance conform to the desired occlusal and aesthetic form, the images can be used with a high degree of confidence to guide implant placement.

8-9 COPYING ANTERIOR GUIDANCE

The problems that may occur when introducing excursive contacts that are not in harmony with the other guidance teeth, the condylar movements and musculature are outlined in Chapter 2. Just to recap, these include pain, decementing and fractured crowns, localised wear, tooth mobility, tooth migration and TMDs. Furthermore, an incorrectly shaped palatal surface may also result in phonetic problems. When a restoration is being provided that includes a guiding surface for mandibular excursions – lateral, protrusive or movements in between – the technician needs to know what form the contacting surface is to take.

Fortunately, technicians are often able to use the adjacent teeth to determine the guidance of a new restoration. For example, if two upper central incisors are being crowned, with all four upper incisors involved in protrusion, then the lateral incisors can be used to dictate the correct guidance on the new crowns. In such cases, the new functional surfaces are relatively straightforward to achieve on a semi-adjustable articulator, or even at the chair-side.

However, if several teeth are to be prepared there may be no existing guiding surfaces left intact after preparation. Under such circumstances, all clues to guidance are lost (Fig 8-46). Where satisfactory guidance is present before preparation, there are several ways of copying it into the definitive restorations. Perhaps the simplest method is to use a putty matrix formed over a cast of the tooth surfaces to be copied. However, reseating the matrix onto a different working cast is error prone and not really appropriate for such precision work.

The two most effective methods to address this problem necessitate the use of a facebow and a semi-adjustable or average value articulator to allow anatomical movements in excursions. These are the "crown-about" method and the "custom incisal guide table" technique.

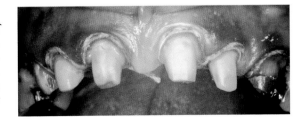

Fig 8-46 Preparation of the anterior teeth has resulted in loss of all the existing guidance surfaces. It is important to plan how to manage this *before* the impressions stage!

141

The Crown-about Method

The simplest way of using this approach is to prepare and fit crowns on alternate teeth. In this way, the technician can copy the guidance from the adjacent unprepared teeth before they, in turn, are prepared. This "every other tooth" method works well where teeth in group function need to be prepared in an upper posterior sextant. You can also use this method for upper anterior restorations, but here technicians prefer to make all the crowns at the same time to optimise aesthetics. In the classic situation where six upper anterior teeth are to be crowned, you will need two impressions:
- an initial impression after preparing every other tooth
- a second impression recorded after the remaining three teeth have been prepared.

In the laboratory, the technician:
1. Makes full-contour wax-ups on the cast from the first impression using the adjacent teeth to inform the shape of the lingual guidance surfaces.
2. Transfers these wax-ups to the second cast to guide the contouring of the three remaining crowns.

The Custom Incisal Guide Table

This method also copies existing guidance. In addition, and unlike the previous method, it enables the guidance to be copied for just one restoration, for example canine guidance in an occlusally sensitive individual in whom you want to minimise any unplanned occlusal changes. It is especially useful when changing anterior guidance using provisional restorations to test that the new shape is satisfactory. The proposed new shape is fashioned using a diagnostic wax-up, as described in Section 8-8.

To make a custom incisal guide table you need, before preparation:
- accurate impressions of the upper and lower teeth or of the provisional crowns to be copied
- a facebow record and a record of ICP if it is not well defined.

Once you have prepared the teeth, record:
- a working impression of all the preparations
- interocclusal records for mounting.

In the laboratory, the technician will:
1. Mount the upper cast of the unprepared teeth on a semi-adjustable or

average value articulator using the facebow record. Mount the lower cast in ICP.

2. Lift the incisal pin by 1 mm, smear it with petroleum jelly, apply a mound of unset acrylic to the incisal table and mould it with the end of the pin during excursions of the articulator until set (Fig 8-47).

3. Check with articulating foil for simultaneous contact between opposing teeth and between pin and custom table.

4. Replace the upper cast with the working cast of the preparation dies.

5. Shape the palatal surfaces of the restorations in accordance with the movements guided by the custom acrylic table (Figs 8-48 and 8-49).

This is an excellent technique, but errors occur if the articulated casts do not follow the true guidance surfaces. Typically, a posterior interference that is not present in the mouth may show up on the articulator as an anomaly. To avoid this problem, the technician may either steepen the condylar guidance to disclude the interference or, preferably after consulting the clinician, the technician may grind the interference off the casts.

The extra effort involved in using these techniques to copy guidance is not enormous. Where several anterior teeth are to be crowned, it is strongly recommended that one of them is used. The articulator is an essential tool in managing anterior guidance and a prerequisite when using guidance copying techniques.

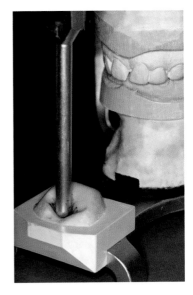

Fig 8-47 To enable tooth guidance to be copied from previously satisfactory surfaces or trial provisional restorations, mount casts that include these surfaces using a facebow and produce a custom incisal guide table.

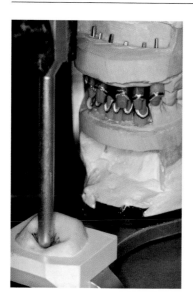

Fig 8-48 The diagnostic casts are replaced with the working casts. In this case the lower crowns are made first, before forming the guidance surfaces in the upper crowns.

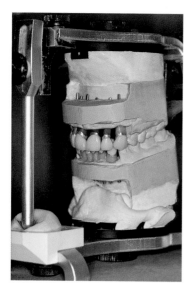

Fig 8-49 Definitive restorations produced using the guide table to conform precisely to the pre-existing guidance.

8-10 STABILISATION SPLINTS

The aim of this section is to consider the uses, construction and adjustment of stabilisation (sometimes spelt "stabilization") splints. These splints, which are an important part of the occlusal management armamentarium, have a wide range of uses, including:

- control of bruxism and associated wear
- management of TMDs
- testing the effect of increasing the occlusal vertical dimension
- splinting mobile teeth affected by reduced periodontal support and heavy, laterally directed occlusal forces.

Whether made for the upper (Fig 8-50) or lower jaw, the purpose of the splint is to incorporate the features of an ideal occlusion. These features include multiple even contacts on the retruded arc of closure, canine guidance with disclusion of the posterior teeth in lateral excursions, and either incisal or canine guidance in protrusion. All these features are included to establish occlusal control.

The anterior guidance ramp should be concave in the upper splint and convex in the lower – similar to the shapes of the tooth guiding surfaces covered by the splint. Upper splints should be used where possible. In patients with a Class III incisor relationship there is often insufficient overjet to support an upper guidance ramp, so a lower splint is better. Canine guidance is not always possible. In such circumstances, guidance ramps should be provided in the premolar regions.

Impressions and Jaw Registration

An accurate impression is critical to the correct fitting of a hard splint. Alginates are adequate for the purpose, but some operators prefer to use addition silicones.

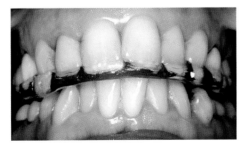

Fig 8-50 Upper stabilisation splint.

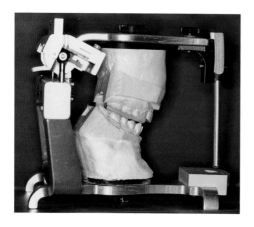

Fig 8-51 Casts mounted in CR on a semi-adjustable articulator. Many technicians use average value instruments with no facebow for splint construction. Opening the articulator gives 2 mm clearance posteriorly.

With splints, the key to successful jaw registration is to record CR at the thickness of the intended splint (Fig 8-51). As the articulator then requires little or no adjustment to the vertical dimension, the casts can be mounted on an average value instrument without the need for a facebow transfer. Splints made in this way usually need only minimal occlusal adjustment when fitted.

Laboratory Procedure

Splints made of heat-cured acrylic are generally stronger and more hygienic than splints of other materials, particularly if the splint has to be worn for a protracted period.

The master cast is mounted and undercuts, including gingival margins, are blocked out or relieved. The technician then duplicates the master cast, draws an outline of the splint in pencil (Fig 8-52) and waxes-up the splint (Fig 8-53). Clasps are not generally needed. Retention can usually be obtained by running the splint over onto the buccal surfaces of the teeth by approximately 1 mm. The wax-up is transferred to the duplicate cast for processing. The processed splint is fitted back onto the master cast to allow fit and occlusion to be refined before return to the clinic.

Splint Fitting

Before looking at the occlusion of the splint, you need to ensure that it is fully seated. At this stage, you will be checking stability, retention and tight-

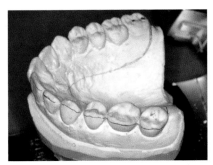

Fig 8-52 Planning of an upper splint. Note the boundaries extending 1–1.5 mm over the buccal aspects of the teeth and the horseshoe-shaped palatal coverage.

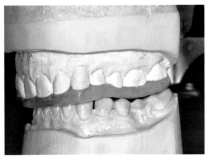

Fig 8-53 A waxed upper splint. Note the flat occlusal surface posteriorly and the guidance ramp anteriorly.

ness as well as seating. In the case of a major discrepancy, do not waste more than 20 minutes fitting the splint; it is likely that you will need either to remake or reline it.

In adjusting the splint's occlusion, it is important to have a mental picture of how the final item should look (Fig 8-54). Your first aim is to eliminate any premature or deflective contacts, such that the opposing teeth hinge straight onto a flat surface. Adjust the splint with the patient in a supine position, to spread single points of contact equally around all opposing teeth, with slightly lighter contacts anteriorly. When it is impossible to obtain an even pattern of contact without excessive grinding, you may decide to make localised additions to the occlusal surface with self-cure acrylic. Beware of creating too thin an occlusal surface; this is likely to perforate or fracture, resulting in loss of occlusal control and overeruption. This stage is usually the one that takes most time.

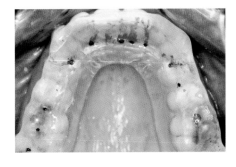

Fig 8-54 Lateral and protrusive guidance ramps showing articulation marks. These are straight, continuous and smooth.

Next, adjust the excursive contacts, checking that the guidance ramps are doing their jobs. Interferences should be removed in the following order: non-working side, then working side and finally protrusive interferences. When removing the interference, it is important to maintain the holding contact marked with black articulating foil. When refining the guidance ramps, check that they are not too steep. The inclines need only be sufficient to give posterior disclusion.

Finally, check the splint with the patient in the upright position. When sitting upright, the patient may notice slightly heavier contacts anteriorly. If present, these should be adjusted. Smooth any rough edges and surfaces using a large rubber cone, or preferably a polishing lathe.

Prescribing Splint Wear

Prescribe night-time wear for nocturnal parafunction and TMDs with symptoms that are worse on waking. Full-time wear is more difficult for the patient, as it may affect both aesthetics and speech. Full-time wear, or at least extended wear, is recommended for patients with TMD pain not obviously related to nocturnal parafunction, in cases when an increase in vertical dimension is being tested, and for patients with increased tooth mobility (periodontal disease having been controlled prior to the provision of the splint).

Not surprisingly, patients often ask how long they need to wear the splint. The following guidance is suggested:
- **For TMDs:** from 3 to 12 months, with the splint being worn much less frequently by most patients towards the end of treatment (see Chapter 6 for advice regarding frequency of adjustment).
- **For nocturnal parafunction:** some patients may need to wear the splint indefinitely. Others just need to use it during periods of psychological stress. It is best to think of the splint as a plastic bumper which protects the teeth from damage, rather than a cure for bruxism.
- **For testing an increase in vertical dimension:** a month of comfortable splint wear is usually sufficient.
- **For patients with increased tooth mobility:** mobility should be reduced in 2–4 weeks of full-time splint wear. Thereafter, it may be necessary to plan an occlusal adjustment to eliminate any deflective contacts and interferences.

Finally, and of great importance, remember to give instructions for cleaning and care of the appliance.

8-11 SPACE CREATION FOR RESTORATIONS

Normally, tooth preparation provides adequate space for crowns and other occlusal coverage restorations. In particular for anterior teeth, sufficient space is needed to accommodate the intercuspal contact and the excursive contact (see Chapter 2).

With posterior teeth, a bevel to the functional cusp – lingual upper, buccal lower – also helps to give sufficient clearance to avoid perforations during adjustment or clinical service. In normal circumstances, no extra space creation is necessary.

When restoring the worn dentition there is an additional problem: how to create sufficient space to accommodate restorative material without destroying further tooth tissue. Further occlusal reduction may threaten the pulp, and may leave a very short and unretentive preparation. Another example of the need for space is where there has been overeruption into a space to be restored with a bridge or a denture. Strategies for creating space form an important part of treatment planning and occlusal management in such situations. Various approaches are summarised in Table 8-5.

Space may be created by simply grinding an opposing tooth. Clearly, a limitation of this technique is the potential to cause dentine sensitivity or even pulp exposure. Fortunately, more conservative techniques are available. These include using the Dahl appliance, increasing the vertical dimension and distalisation. The other techniques listed can be useful on occasion. The outdated approach of devitalising a tooth and placing a post with a reangulated core is not recommended. Not only is this approach extremely destructive, the resulting non-axial forces may cause root fracture. This section considers only the three most useful techniques.

Dahl Appliance

This appliance was originally devised in the 1970s as a partial coverage bite plane made of cobalt chrome. It was prescribed in patients with localised wear of the lingual surfaces of the upper anterior teeth to create space through a combination of intrusion of the anterior teeth and dentoalveolar extrusion of the posteriors. The appliance is shaped to provide axial loading of the opposing teeth and smooth guidance in excursions. It is very effective in the majority of patients, but it can take several months to obtain sufficient space (1–2 mm) for a crown or adhesively retained restoration.

Table 8-5 **Space creation strategies for restorations** (continued over page)

Strategy	Indications	Advantages	Disadvantages
Grind opposing tooth	Single or small number of teeth requiring slight adjustment	Simple	Dentine exposure: sensitivity, discolouration Adjustment limited
Dahl appliance	Localised wear of lingual surfaces of maxillary anterior teeth Posterior tooth erupted into bounded edentulous space	No tooth destruction 2–3 mm of space can be obtained	Tooth movements take several months Occasionally does not work
Increase vertical dimension	Generalised wear necessitating longer crowns for aesthetics and improved retention	Full axial wall length of preparation can be maintained	All teeth in one or both arches may need occlusal coverage
Distalisation	Localised wear of lingual surfaces of maxillary teeth	No anterior tooth reduction needed	Limited to cases with large horizontal component of RCP–ICP slide Need for posterior tooth occlusal adjustment
Crown lengthening	May be used for localised and generalised wear problems, often in combination with one of the other techniques	Simple if electrosurgery can be used Retention augmented by increased axial wall height	Bone removal likely to be needed if no pocketing present
Orthodontics	Very occasionally used to increase overjet or improve alignment of anterior segment	Limits tooth destruction	Classical orthodontics not good for producing dentoalveolar intrusion

Table 8-5 **Space creation strategies for restorations** (continued)

Strategy	Indications	Advantages	Disadvantages
Devitalisation with post and core	Popular for localised space problems before Dahl appliance introduced	None – unless tooth requires endodontic treatment anyway	Realignment of core in combination with RCT can put tooth at risk of fracture
Surgical repositioning	Often a sledgehammer to crack a nut	May limit tooth destruction and allows correction of concomitant skeletal and dentoalveolar discrepancies	Surgical morbidity

The original removable version sometimes suffered poor patient compliance. As a result, fixed versions of the Dahl appliance were devised, made from composite (Fig 8-55) or nickel chrome cemented with a glass–ionomer cement (Fig 8-56). Cementation of the cast-metal version with glass–ionomer cement allows the appliance to be removed relatively easily. Provided there are no retentive features in the tooth preparation, a slot is simply created at the margin and an instrument inserted and twisted to break the lute.

The Dahl approach is a form of orthodontic treatment. As such, patients need to be carefully informed of what to expect, in particular the change in sensation experienced when eating with the posterior teeth out of occlusion. Patients need to know that they are unlikely to have posterior occlusion for perhaps 3–6 months. The movement can occur rapidly, on occasion in as little as 6–8 weeks, so early review is essential. It is unusual for the teeth not to move at all, given time. However, this is a recognised problem and may require an alternative strategy, for example adhesive onlays or long-term review, if the patient is not concerned by the lack of contact. In other words, have a "plan B".

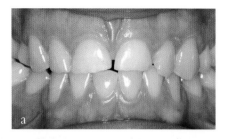

Fig 8-55 Composite Dahl appliance.

Fig 8-55a Patient with worn central incisors caused by parafunctional tooth grinding.

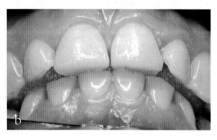

Fig 8-55b Composite built onto lingual surfaces of the central incisors to increase the vertical dimension by 1.5 mm – notice how the other teeth are lifted out of occlusion by the pronounced cingulum contours.

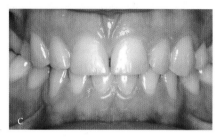

Fig 8-55c After 4 months the posterior teeth re-established occlusion, but unusually the daytime parafunction restarted and some posterior occlusal adjustment was needed to improve occlusal comfort.

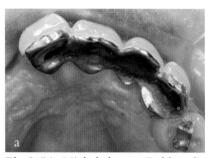
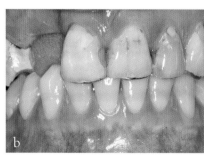

Fig 8-56 Nickel chrome Dahl appliance.
(a) Viewed palatally, the pronounced cingulum table is designed to cause axial loading of the upper and lower anterior teeth. (b) The appliance extends up to the incisal edges and is secured with glass–ionomer cement. At three months the posterior teeth have almost regained contact.

Surprisingly, most patients cope with all forms of Dahl appliance very well, including those on posterior teeth. The localised build-up to increase vertical dimension has not been reported to aggravate or precipitate TMD; however, caution must be exercised in TMD patients. As always, treat the TMD first. As the back teeth re-establish contact, patients may experience some discomfort from occlusal interferences. This is unusual, but it can be relieved through minor occlusal adjustment.

A recent development is the use of the Dahl approach to reverse the overeruption of molars into opposing edentulous spaces as a prelude to the provision of definitive bridgework (Fig 8-57).

Another is to make the definitive restoration to the required thickness, so it acts as its own Dahl appliance. With the development of modern composites, anterior teeth can be built up directly, but one should be vigilant for wear of the material. This same approach has been recommended for adhesive bridges, with thickened retainers (0.7 mm rather than 0.5 mm), extending onto the incisal edges without any occlusal reduction. Such retainers are rigid, theoretically reducing stresses in the resin lute. This should in turn lower the risk of debond. This seems an attractive proposition, but care is required to arrange the occlusal stops and anterior guidance to maintain occlusal control. Often, a fixed–fixed design of bridge is needed, otherwise unwanted pontic movement may occur – a possible problem with a single-retainer cantilever bridge subject to excursive contact on its pontic (see Section 8-12).

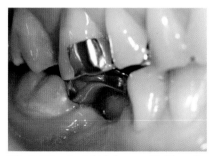

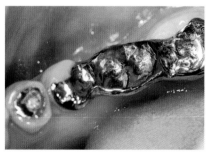

Fig 8-57a A nickel chrome Dahl appliance designed as an arched pontic, used to reverse the overeruption of the upper right first molar.

Fig 8-57b Occlusal view. This patient, treated by Dr Paul King, had similar appliances bilaterally and found them reasonably comfortable to wear. Intrusion of the upper first molars took 9 months.

The Dahl approach is an excellent, scientifically supported and conservative method of space creation. It should be used as an alternative to a general increase in vertical dimension, and helps avoid unnecessary tooth preparation. Reversal of overerupted posterior teeth and supraoccluding adhesive bridgework are promising applications not yet supported by comprehensive clinical trial data. As with any treatment not supported by good evidence, patients should be apprised of the relatively untried nature of such treatment before being asked to give consent.

Increasing Vertical Dimension

An increase in vertical dimension means restoring all the occlusal surfaces of one or both arches to obtain a stable pattern of occlusal contact. This is clearly a major undertaking, requiring meticulous planning and the use of appropriate planning aids, such as mounted casts and wax-ups. The principles of such a reorganisation are covered in detail in Chapter 4.

The purpose of a change in vertical dimension is often to create space anteriorly for aesthetic restorations in wear cases, allowing the teeth to be restored to a more natural length. Anterior wear is often accompanied by posterior wear, and increasing the vertical dimension allows this problem to be addressed simultaneously. Worn teeth are often short occlusogingivally, offering limited crown height (critical to crown retention). Occlusal clearance is achieved through jaw opening, removing or reducing the need for further occlusal reduction (Fig 8-58). This approach is extremely useful in cases in which the worn posterior teeth require full-coverage restorations, or when exposed dentine is sensitive and needs to be covered by adhesively retained onlays.

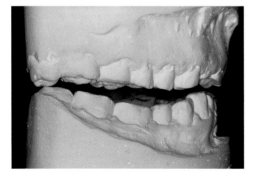

Fig 8-58 Increasing vertical dimension. The patient was suffering with generalised wear, which was more severe anteriorly. A full-mouth reconstruction was prescribed, with a 4 mm increase in vertical dimension, to provide space for anterior restorations. This approach had the advantage that no occlusal reduction was needed in the preparations of the posterior teeth for crowns.

Increasing vertical dimension may also create space for denture connectors and saddles. However, in adopting such an approach, a stable occlusion must be provided by the remaining teeth. If occlusal stability relies on the patient wearing partial dentures, problems may arise if for any reason dentures cannot be worn.

The traditional approach to increasing vertical dimension involves first testing the increase with a stabilisation splint (see Section 8-10). The splint may then be used as a platform to maintain occlusal stability while groups of teeth are restored. As new restorations are fitted, the splint can be cut away and relined with self-cure acrylic to maintain retention and stability. A more immediate approach, using adhesively retained restorations to create the increase in vertical dimension without an initial period of splint wear, is gaining popularity. Clinical experience shows this to be successful. It makes sense, however, to use a period of initial splint wear to test a patient's compliance in cases where the final restorations will need to be protected from destructive nocturnal parafunction by means of a splint. An increase in vertical dimension should not be trialled with a tissue-borne partial denture as this will cause trauma to the denture-bearing areas.

At some point in the treatment, the new vertical dimension has to be established, whether or not a splint is used. The step that makes the change permanent is the most important and difficult one. It is recommended that the teeth are built up strategically to the required vertical dimension, often using directly placed composite. Cores or provisional restorations may also be used. If the treatment has been planned using a diagnostic wax-up – the preferred technique – the final result can be visualised and matrices formed to facilitate the provision of direct composite or provisional restorations.

A good place to start is the lower incisors, if they need to be increased in length. Adhesive dentistry is always preferable in such situations, as the preparation of lower incisors is very destructive. Next, the upper incisors can be built up with either composite or provisional restorations, taking care to establish stable ICP stops and harmonious anterior guidance. At this stage, the posterior teeth will be lifted out of contact and the new vertical dimension established. If left in this relationship for more than a few days, the Dahl effect will start to take place. Therefore, it is important to build up the posterior teeth without too much delay, otherwise occlusal space will be lost. Again, adhesive composite can be used as an interim material or, alternatively, a strong glass–ionomer (e.g. Fuji IX), which has the benefit of being easily and quickly applied. Metal shims are especially useful and are an efficient means of restoring the posterior occlusion where the teeth are worn but otherwise unrestored. Porcelain shims are a good option for patients without parafunction and with sufficient space (> 1.5 mm). Once anterior guidance and posterior stability have been achieved, definitive crowns can be provided.

Distalisation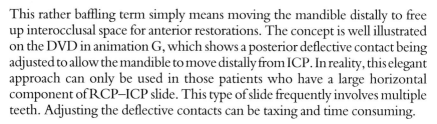

This rather baffling term simply means moving the mandible distally to free up interocclusal space for anterior restorations. The concept is well illustrated on the DVD in animation G, which shows a posterior deflective contact being adjusted to allow the mandible to move distally from ICP. In reality, this elegant approach can only be used in those patients who have a large horizontal component of RCP–ICP slide. This type of slide frequently involves multiple teeth. Adjusting the deflective contacts can be taxing and time consuming.

However, where it can be used, it is an extremely attractive solution, as it obviates the need for increasing the vertical dimension, which is just as taxing and much more time consuming. Distalising is worth considering if the anterior teeth show signs of fremitus resulting from posterior deflective contacts causing an anterior thrust. Simultaneous equilibration has the double benefit of creating space and reducing adverse loading on new restorations (Fig 8-59).

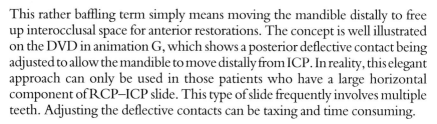

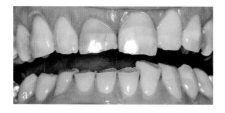

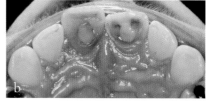

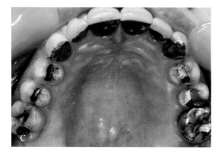

Fig 8-59 Distalisation of the mandible. (a) Patient with worn and traumatised incisors. (b) Upper incisors viewed palatally. (c) To make space for anterior restorations, the posterior teeth were equilibrated to eliminate a large RCP–ICP slide with a mainly horizontal component. The bur marks on the premolars remain to be smoothed and polished.

8-12 ADJUSTING NEW RESTORATIONS

Procedural inaccuracies and overeruption often conspire to make well-fitting restoration "high" when returned from the laboratory. To assess how much adjustment is needed, it is best to remove the restoration and identify, using shim stock, a pair of adjacent occluding teeth, termed "index teeth". After reseating the restoration, the index teeth will be lifted out of occlusion, giving a visual indication of the amount of adjustment needed.

Visually checking the occlusion gives only an indication of the amount of adjustment needed. Articulating foils, and preferably shim stock, give quantification (see Section 8-1). Some articulating papers resemble blotting paper in consistency and thickness; such papers are prone to leaving false marks, and they may even alter the patient's position of closure. Some articulating papers can be as thick as 200 μm. This is over ten times as thick as the best foils, which are infinitely preferable. Despite their higher cost, the accuracy and precision with which foils mark a restoration can save a great deal of time and effort, provided the teeth are dry. Marking of metal occlusal surfaces is much easier if technicians lightly sandblast or glass bead them before delivery. When doing this, the technician needs to protect the polish of the axial surfaces with ribbon wax.

Both restoration and adjacent teeth should hold shim stock firmly in ICP (Fig 8-60). However, anterior teeth often have light shim stock contacts which should be kept light after restoration. Failure to achieve this can result in occlusal overload of the restored or opposing tooth, which in turn can cause pain, mobility, fracture or displacement.

In addition to using shim stock and articulating foils, it is worth listening to the occlusion with and without the crown in place. You can readily hear occlusal discrepancies when patients tap their teeth together.

A large flame-shaped diamond in a high-speed or speed-increasing handpiece should be used for occlusal adjustment. It may occasionally be necessary to adjust the tooth opposing a restoration to avoid crown perforation or exposure of rough opaque porcelain. Such adjustments should be planned with the patient's consent. A thickness gauge, for example a Svensen gauge, is invaluable for predicting areas vulnerable to perforation (Fig 8-61).

If you take proper notice of the occlusion during preparation, however, the risk of perforation should be minimal.

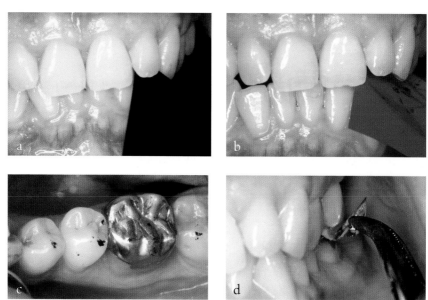

Fig 8-60 Occlusal adjustment of a new posterior restoration.
(a) Even contacts established in ICP using black articulating foil. (b) Excursions checked with red foil. In this case, the non-working side is being checked for interferences. (c) A stable pattern of ICP holding contacts with disclusion in all excursions and no deflective contacts. (d) Shim stock is used to check the firmness of occlusal contacts in comparison with those on the selected index teeth.

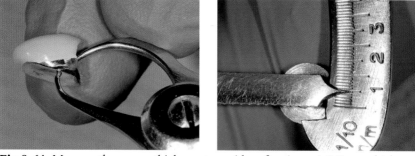

Fig 8-61 Measure the crown thickness to avoid perforations. A 0.5 mm thickness is a minimum requirement anteriorly and 1 mm posteriorly.

Once ICP has been re-established, the excursions can be checked, preferably using a different coloured foil, typically red. ICP contacts are then re-marked over the top of the initial marks using the original colour, normally black, allowing the excursive contact to be differentiated and refined. The decision about whether the restoration is to be involved in guiding jaw movement (generally with anterior teeth) or whether there should be disclusion (as often occurs posteriorly) should have been made well before this stage. Finally, it is worth guiding back the mandible into the retruded path of closure to ensure the restoration is not introducing a new deflective contact.

When constructing multiple anterior crowns, the technician can ensure a satisfactory pattern of excursive contact (Fig 8-62), avoiding or reducing loading of the weak lateral incisors – assuming that a suitable articulator and guidance copying (as described in Section 8-9) have been used. With cantilever bridges, especially those having only a single abutment, it is important to ensure the pontic is not loaded in excursions (Fig 8-63).

With veneers, it is easy to be lulled into a false sense of security. Being cemented to the buccal aspect of teeth, veneers seem immune to occlusal considerations. However, a veneer taken over the incisal edge has the potential to interfere with excursions and can be prone to fracture or damage. Moreover, a bulky veneer may interfere in an eccentric excursion in which the lower incisors cross over the upper incisal edges. "Giant teeth", associated with certain aesthetic techniques, can markedly increase tooth length. This requires care with both guidance and the crossover onto the buccal side of the veneer.

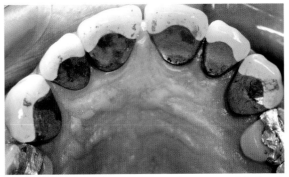

Fig 8-62 Occlusal adjustment of six upper anterior crowns. Notice that each crown has a light ICP holding contact (*marked in black*). Excursive contacts (*marked in red*) can be sited either on the marginal ridges or more centrally. The lateral excursions are canine guided, while protrusion is guided principally by the central incisors.

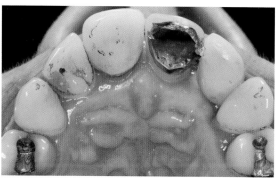

Fig 8-63 Occlusal adjustment of an adhesive cantilever bridge replacing the upper left lateral incisor (mirror shot). Notice that the pontic has a light ICP holding contact to prevent overeruption, but is free from any excursive contact. There is a risk of causing excessive mobility, drifting or dislodging the bridge if the pontic is loaded in excursions.

If restorations do not make occlusal contact, it may be acceptable just to monitor them and adjust interferences as necessary. Should they cause discomfort or occlusal instability, they may need to be remade. If in doubt, cement them with soft cement to facilitate subsequent removal.

The overwhelming message is that if all the preceding stages have been properly executed it should not be necessary to make any more than minor adjustments.

Finishing and Polishing

The final stage prior to cementation is polishing. A rough surface, especially in porcelain, will rapidly wear the opposing tooth. Therefore it is very important to use a sequence of abrasives designed for the material in question to achieve a smooth surface or to reglaze the restoration. Adjusted metal surfaces can be finished with finishing burs followed by rubber abrasive points. Abrasive discs are useful for flat areas, such as proximal contact areas, and can be used on either metal or porcelain. Porcelain can also be finished using composite finishing diamonds, but a light touch and water spray are needed to avoid stripping off the diamond coating. Further finishing is achieved with white rubber abrasive points followed by a felt wheel or by a rubber cup charged with diamond polishing paste. Alternatively, a metal ceramic crown can be reglazed as can some types of all-ceramic crown.

Follow-up

Sometimes, even a well-adjusted occlusion can change with time. While changes may be inconsequential, they can result in damaging prematurities, deflective contacts and interferences. Monitoring is therefore recommended. Such monitoring can be as simple as checking shim contacts and feeling around for fremitus when the teeth are tapped together. In addition, check your restorations for signs of damage from parafunction, including marked faceting and chipping of porcelain. Depending on the findings, some minor occlusal adjustment or the fitting of a splint may be indicated.

Further Reading

The glossary of prosthodontic terms. J Prosthet Dent 2005;94(1):10–92.

Ibbetson R. Clinical considerations for adhesive bridgework. Dental Update 2004;31:254–256, 258, 260 passim.

Jagger RG, Korszun A. Phantom bite revisited. Br Dent J 2004;197:241–243.

Moufti MA, Lillico JT, Wassell RW. How to make a well-fitting stabilization splint. Dent Update 2007;34:398-408.

Pameijer JN. Periodontal and occlusal factors in crown and bridge procedures. Dental Centre for Postgraduate Courses; Amsterdam, 1985.

Potts M, Prata N, Walsh J, Grossman A. Parachute approach to evidence based medicine. BMJ 2006;333:701–703.

Poyser NJ, Porter RW, Briggs PF, Chana HS, Kelleher MG. The Dahl concept: past, present and future. Br Dent J 2005;198:669–676; quiz 720.

Redman CD, Hemmings KW, Good JA. The survival and clinical performance of resin-based composite restorations used to treat localised anterior tooth wear. Br Dent J 2003;194:566–572; discussion 559.

Shillingburg HT, Hobo S, Whitsett LD et al. (1997) Fundamentals of Fixed Prosthodontics. 3rd edn. Chicago: Quintessence, 1997:335-354.

Smith GC, Pell JP. Parachute use to prevent death and major trauma related to gravitational challenge: systematic review of randomised controlled trials. BMJ 2003;327(7429):1459–1461.

Tupac RG. Clinical importance of voluntary and induced Bennett movement. J Prosthet Dent 1978;40:39–43.

Index

Quintessentials for General Dental Practitioners Series

in 44 volumes

Editor-in-Chief: Professor Nairn H F Wilson

The Quintessentials for General Dental Practitioners Series covers basic principles and key issues in all aspects of modern dental medicine. Each book can be read as a stand-alone volume or in conjunction with other books in the series.

Publication date, approximately

Clinical Practice, Editor: Nairn Wilson

Culturally Sensitive Oral Healthcare	available
Dental Erosion	available
Special Care Dentistry	available
Evidence-based Dentistry	available
Infection Control for the Dental Team	Summer 2008

Oral Surgery and Oral Medicine, Editor: John G Meechan

Practical Dental Local Anaesthesia	available
Practical Oral Medicine	available
Practical Conscious Sedation	available
Minor Oral Surgery in Dental Practice	available

Imaging, Editor: Keith Horner

Interpreting Dental Radiographs	available
Panoramic Radiology	available
21st Century Dental Imaging	available

Periodontology, Editor: Iain L C Chapple

Understanding Periodontal Diseases: Assessment and Diagnostic Procedures in Practice	available
Decision-Making for the Periodontal Team	available
Successful Periodontal Therapy – A Non-Surgical Approach	available
Periodontal Management of Children, Adolescents and Young Adults	available
Periodontal Medicine: A Window on the Body	available
Contemporary Periodontal Surgery – An Illustrated Guide to the Art Behind the Science	available

Endodontics, Editor: John M Whitworth

Rational Root Canal Treatment in Practice	available
Managing Endodontic Failure in Practice	available
Adhesive Restoration of Endodontically Treated Teeth	available

Prosthodontics, Editor: P Finbarr Allen

Teeth for Life for Older Adults	available
Complete Dentures – from Planning to Problem Solving	available
Removable Partial Dentures	available
Fixed Prosthodontics in Dental Practice	available
Applied Occlusion	available
Orofacial Pain: A Guide for General Practitioners	available

Operative Dentistry, Editor: Paul A Brunton

Decision-Making in Operative Dentistry	available
Aesthetic Dentistry	available
Communicating in Dental Practice	available
Indirect Restorations	available
Dental Bleaching	available
Dental Materials in Operative Dentistry	available
Successful Posterior Composites	available

Paediatric Dentistry/Orthodontics, Editor: Marie Therese Hosey

Child Taming: How to Manage Children in Dental Practice	available
Paediatric Cariology	available
Treatment Planning for the Developing Dentition	available
Managing Dental Trauma in Practice	available

General Dentistry and Practice Management, Editor: Raj Rattan

The Business of Dentistry	available
Risk Management in General Dental Practice	available
Quality Matters: From Clinical Care to Customer Service	available

Dental Team, Editor: Mabel Slater

Team Players in Dentistry	Summer 2008

Implantology, Editor: Lloyd J Searson

Implantology in General Dental Practice	available

Quintessence Publishing Co. Ltd., London